Ebola Diaries

Six weeks to save the world

Dr John Wright

For Katherine, Megan and Ciara
My Three Graces

All proceeds from the sale of this book are donated to the Against Malaria Foundation who provide simple bed nets to help protect children and parents from malaria
www.againstmalaria.com

Forward

An epidemic that took the world by surprise. A simple RNA virus that started in bats and spread to humans. It began slowly and then gathered pace with exponential speed. Governments were complacent and slow to act, but eventually they shut borders, closed schools and businesses, cancelled football matches. Society was transformed by fear: no more hugging or touching, obsessive hand washing and hypochondriasis.

Health care workers became the canaries in the mine – the first to catch and spread the infection. Hospital and health care centres became amplification centres for transmission and naturally the people stayed away. The health care workers became heroes but also lepers as communities began worry that they were germ spreaders.

There were endless debates about PPE with guidance that changed weekly. Health care workers stepped nervously into red zone wards, never having been so scared in their professional lives, but with incredible resilience adapted to their new surroundings with speed and confidence. Scientists raced to find a vaccine.

This was not covid. This was the Ebola epidemic in 2014. I was one of the first NHS volunteers to go out to Sierra Leone where I worked with the British Army to set up an Ebola Treatment Centre and then run it and support the wider public health response in a rural community 6 hours from the capital of

Freetown. This diary tells the inside story of my work as a doctor on the Ebola frontline as I travel from my safe European home to the eye of the storm, working with the British army to set up and run an Ebola Treatment Centre and coordinating a public health emergency response in one of the poorest places in the world. Told with humour and honesty, it provides a real-time record of one of the biggest global threats to health in recent years.

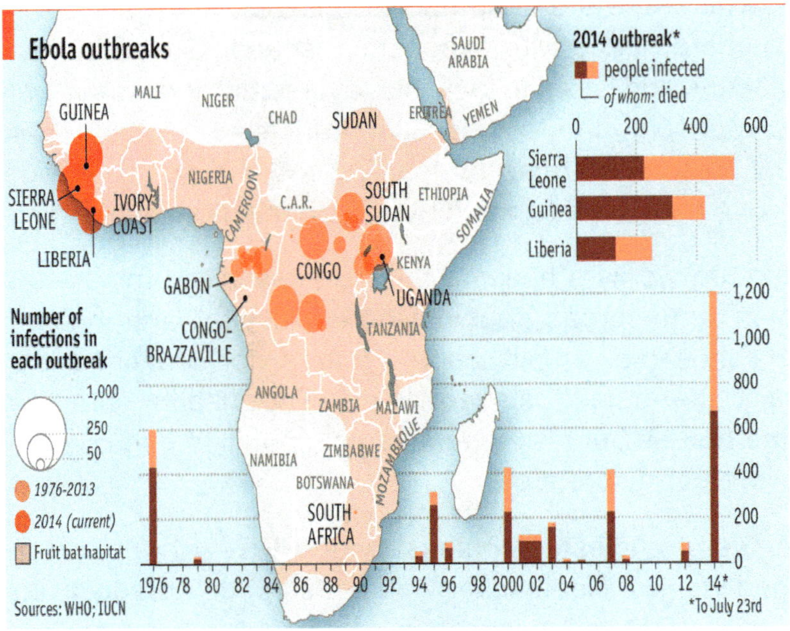

BBC Diaries

During my journey I recorded a series for the BBC from my army barracks training through to my return one year after the epidemic. The audio diaries capture the voices of my clinical colleagues, village chiefs, radio DJs and worried families and will bring to life the written diaries.

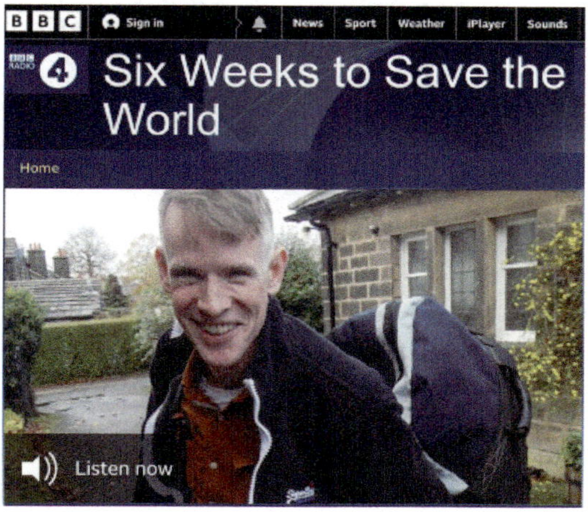

https://www.bbc.co.uk/programmes/b04vdnbq

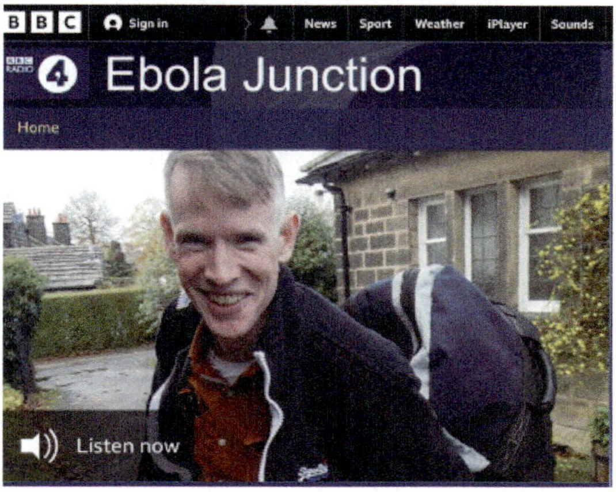

https://www.bbc.co.uk/programmes/b053749b

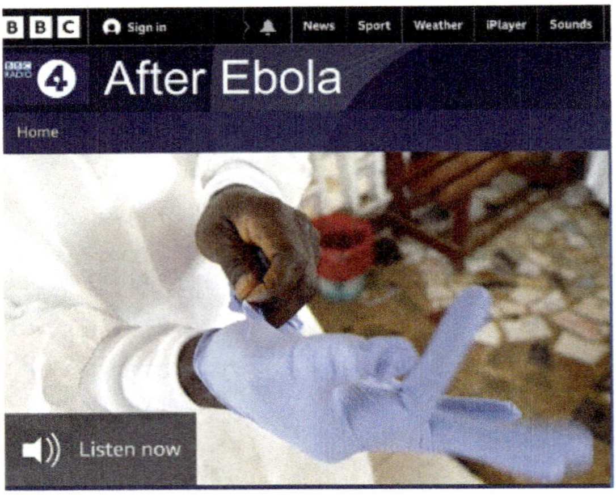

]https://www.bbc.co.uk/programmes/b06tr5t5

Prelude

On the 2nd December 2013 Emile Ouamouno fell ill with a fever. He lived in the remote village of Meliandou in Guinea and used to play in a tree near his house where fruit bats roosted. Four days later he was dead. Emile was case zero in what was to become one of the greatest threats to global health in a generation, killing thousands of people and triggering an international red alert.

A few days after his death his sister fell ill. Then his mother. Then his grandmother. A nurse who had attended Emile carried the deadly virus back to the health centre before falling sick and dying. Before she died she had infected her healthcare colleagues who carried the deadly virus home to their families and away to neighbouring villages.

It had begun, yet tragically no one would know until over three months later when in March 2014 the WHO reported the first cases of Ebola in West Africa. By this time the evil genie was well out of his bottle, moving from village to town and from town to city, and from city to country, hitchhiking on a broken public health network. The virus, named after a white water river where is was first identified in 1976 in the Democratic Republic of Congo, had not been found in West Africa before. Soon it would cast a long and terrifying shadow.

In May 2014 a group of family and friends travelled across the Eastern border from Sierra Leone to Guinea to attend a funeral of a traditional healer. Like the healthcare workers the healer had been trying to cure Ebola cases. Ebola is most infectious shortly after death, a cunning evolutionary trick that would aid its spread in West Africa where the bodies of recently deceased are held closely and kissed with parting affection as part of mourning rituals.

By the end of May the first cases in Sierra Leone were reported - increasing slowly and then exponentially. In Kenema when the epidemic first arrived, the hospital had one of the world's only Lassa fever isolation units, with clinicians who were experts in dealing with a hemorrhagic fever very similar to Ebola. Yet within weeks the local health care system was overwhelmed. 23 out of the 24 nurses working at the hospital were infected with Ebola, and 12 of them died, as did the country's only experienced infectious disease doctor Dr Sheik Khan, the ambulance drivers and lab technicians. This was the health service's Chernobyl for the Ebola epidemic.

By July the first cases were reported in the capital Freetown. Urgent public health campaigns were launched and in August a state of emergency was declared, however the Ebola horse had well and truly bolted. By October hospitals had run out of beds and supplies and burial teams were struggling to keep up with burying the number of bodies. In November the UK government began to build the first of six Ebola Treatment Centres and asked a number of Non-Governmental Organisations to help run them. This is when my story begins.

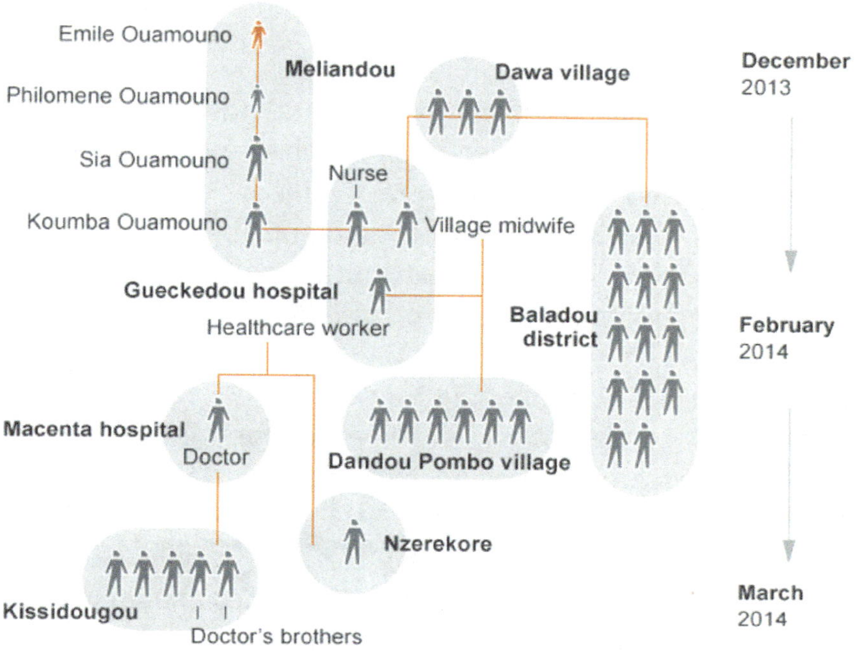

Source: New England Journal of Medicine

Wednesday, 12 November 2014
Six weeks to save the world

Like the rest of the World I had been following the news about the Ebola epidemic with growing concern. The newspaper stories about the rapid spread of this virulent organism, and the television pictures from countries affected showing the human tragedy unfolding had rung internal alarm bells. However, it was a long way away, in a part of the word I was unlikely to ever visit. Then in September a report from the US Centers for Disease Control was published indicating that unless urgent action was taken, the number of cases could mushroom from the current figure of 8,000 to over a million by the start of 2015. The Ebola epidemic had become the biggest global public health threat in modern history and we had just weeks left to save the world.

I have worked in Africa for nearly 25 years. In the early 1990s I was a doctor in a rural African hospital when the new epidemics of TB, cholera and HIV/AIDS hit the continent. Over subsequent years I was able to work with local communities and clinicians in Africa to establish public health programmes to help early identification, treatment and prevention of both TB and HIV/AIDS. Having seen at first hand the human suffering from these epidemics I felt I should put my hand up and offer to help with Ebola, so I googled "UK emergency Ebola response" and ten minutes later had registered to volunteer in Sierra Leone.

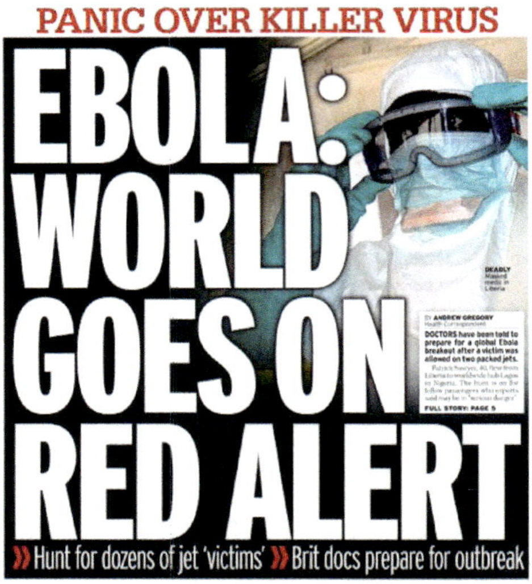
PANIC OVER KILLER VIRUS

EBOLA: WORLD GOES ON RED ALERT

DEADLY Masked medic in Liberia

By ANDREW GREGORY
Health Correspondent

DOCTORS have been told to prepare for a global Ebola breakout after a victim was allowed on two packed jets.

Patrick Sawyer, 40, flew from Liberia to worldwide hub Lagos in Nigeria. The hunt is on for fellow passengers who experts said may be in "serious danger"

FULL STORY: PAGE 5

» Hunt for dozens of jet 'victims' » Brit docs prepare for outbreak

The website informed me that they had been inundated with offers from doctors and nurses in the UK to help and so not to expect a response. Inside I breathed a sigh of relief; I had done my duty by showing willingness to volunteer, but being at the back of the queue for this particular call seemed a safe distance from the fatal clutches of the Ebola virus.

Then two weeks later at 9pm on a Thursday evening I got a call from the Ebola emergency response team to ask if I would join the first wave of NHS clinicians going out to Sierra Leone. There had been over 1000 NHS volunteers, and 30 had been chosen for the first emergency response team. A flicker of flattery about being selected was quickly drowned by a wave of panic as I started to appreciate what I had let myself in for. After a somber late night discussion with my wife, I agreed to go.

Suddenly my life was turned upside down. I had one week's notice before being sent for Ministry of Defence training and then straight out to Freetown and to the heart of this deadly epidemic. I had to get permission from my Medical Director for professional leave, from my Born in Bradford and Improvement Academy colleagues to cover my work and from my clinical colleagues to cover my clinics. I had a week to put my life into deep freeze which was strangely liberating but also illuminating in how quickly I could be replaced!

Over the next few weeks I will attempt to describe this unexpected journey from my safe European home in Bradford to the eye of the storm in Sierra Leone.

Thursday, 13 November 2014
Farewell to Family: I'm in the Army Now

After a day timetabled "Farewell to family" I have packed up my impressively new kitbag and am heading off for Royal Army Medical Services Training. It's a nine day residential training course with the NHS team travelling from across the UK to the Queen Elizabeth Barracks in York. The plan is to fly us out to Sierra Leone on the final day, so we have been told to pack clothes to deal with the cold and wet of Yorkshire as well as the tropical heat of Africa. Lots of dithering about how to manage this combination, but eventually settling on a UK bag and an African bag.

We had a family reunion at the weekend, so it was a serendipitous opportunity to say goodbye to my daughters – wish them Happy Christmas and reassure them that I would take care of myself. We go to a Specials gig and dance together, and join arms to 'You're wondering now, what to do, now you know this is the end' – a hymn to solidarity though I'm not sure it is the note of optimism I would like to leave on.

They are nervous for me, but also proud about their dad which makes me feel a bit of a fraud. My wife is supportive as always, and preparing herself for two months alone in the house – meals for one and the cats for company.

My army marching orders provide precise instructions about booking into camp and what to expect (military food and barracks accommodation). I am advised to bring my PT kit, but I don't think I have one.

The British army are building the Ebola Treatment Centres (ETCs) in Sierra Leone, and providing the rigorous training for health care workers. However the ETCs are being run by non-governmental organisations such as Medecins Sans Frontieres and Save the Children. Our team of 30 have been assigned to each of these, and I have been told I will be joining Medecins Du Monde or Doctors of the World to help set up and run the new ETC in Moyamba.

There are multiple layers involved in the emergency response – from the UK government and DfID, the emergency response recruitment team, the training team, the NGO team in the UK and the NGO team in country. Unsurprisingly for such a rapidly changing emergency there is considerable uncertainty about what is happening and what to expect when we arrive. However each day brings a little more light on the situation.

I'm keen to find out more about what diagnostic tests and what treatments will be available. In the low resource setting in which we will be working these will be extremely limited, but I am surprised to find out that MSF are recommending that no intravenous lines are used on patients in the ETCs. This seems such a basic medical intervention, yet the risk of contamination of health care workers with Ebola infected blood appears to be paramount. So the care provided sounds more palliative than I had expected.

So my bags are packed and it's time to go. Leaving in a Renault Clio today, but the jet plane arrives next week.

Saturday, 15 November 2014
Personal Protection Equipment Training

I adjust to me new army barracks home. As the son of Irish republican parents I have been acculturated with an antipathy towards our armed forces, but find myself warmly welcomed by a young and diverse group of army trainers who give me a sense of pride in our country. Accommodation is basic - small basic beds in a dormitory. No turn down service or chocolates on the pillow.

After two days of briefings about the clinical and political aspects of the Ebola outbreak, we get down to the dress rehearsals. The Personal Protection Equipment (PPE) will be our shield against infection in the Ebola Treatment Centre, and it is the army's job to make sure we can put it on and take it off in our sleep.

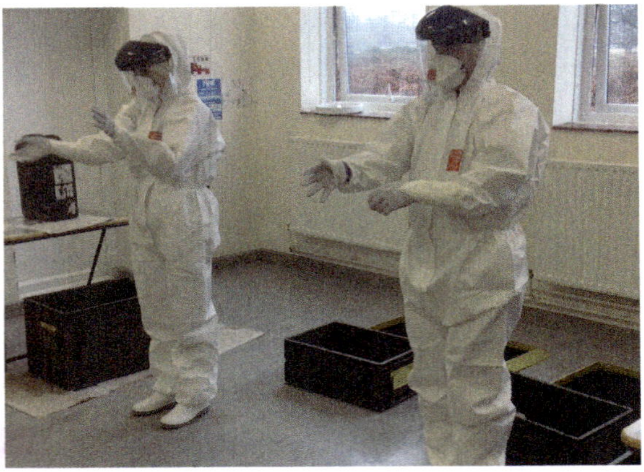

We dress in surgical scrubs, then a high protection gown, then an apron. A hair-net, full face visor and hood, and two pairs of gloves. The donning takes about 10 minutes, teaming up with a buddy and checking each other at every stage to make sure we are fully covered. The checking routines are observed religiously, and our buddy will be a very critical friend as we enter, work in and then leave the Ebola ward.

The doffing of the PPE is the toughest part and takes about 20 minutes. We have to make sure that none of our Ebola contaminated PPE gets anywhere near our skin or face. The exit from the Ebola ward is an assault course of chlorine baths and wash stations. At every stage we work in pairs to remove one item at a time – a life and death Full Monty. Two monitors observe us all the time – shouting to us to stop if we make any mistakes.

WHY CHLORINE
CAN THAT KILL THE VIRUS?

The army does this sort of thing very well. They train all the time for high risk situations with drills and checklists to ensure that all their soldiers do exactly the right thing, all the time. On the walls of our classroom there are mnemonics and reminders reinforcing all the steps needed to shoot an assault rifle or undertake a night mission. This discipline is now applied to preparing the fight against Ebola.

The PPE suits become uncomfortable after about 20 minutes, but this is in a classroom setting on a cold Yorkshire winter's day. Our next stage is to move to full simulation in a purpose-built field hospital that is a replica for the Ebola Treatment Centres the army are busy constructing as we practice. Large field hospital tents surrounded by fencing with public health warnings about Ebola provide our theatre stage. We practice putting IV lines up, taking blood, decontaminating when we get exposed. Every step has been worked through with experts from Porton Down, and there are SOPs for every occasion. There are lots of lessons for improving patient safety in the NHS – checklists, communication, human factors, simulation training.

Even taking a blood sample is a protracted procedure. The blood has to be protected by a plastic bag and the blood tube by a large protective tube, everything sprayed and double sprayed in chlorine and then carried out in a bucket of chlorine.

After training in the PPE suits for an hour it is becoming uncomfortably hot and oppressive. We stop and break, and then move up to 1.5 hours. The relief of doffing the PPE after this time is enormous, but requires the patience of the 20 minutes choreographed decontamination. The temperature in the field hospital is 20 degrees. Tomorrow they turn on the heaters to simulate the summer heat of Sierra Leone.

Sunday, 16 November 2014
Military Training for the Ebola War

The Royal Army Medical Training Centre is the perfect place for our training, with great facilities and enormous experience in biohazards and simulation. The military world is a different sort of universe from mine, with an emphasis on killing people rather than trying to stop them dying. However, the military connection is appropriate for this new Ebola crisis. This is a classic example of a battle between two populations of species – pathogen and host. On the pathogen side there is the Zaire Ebola virus – evolutionary successful at crossing species and highly effective at spreading – at its most infective when the host is just dead, so in the animal world where it normally resides, it can spread quickly when other animals scavenge the warm remains of the last victim. On the host side there are humans as the defending army, poorly prepared for this particular battle through poverty, overcrowding, lack of basic public health defences and with only fragile health services to provide support.

There are 60 Ebola warriors on this first army training test run – 30 from the NHS and 30 from Norway, joining forces in a model of international collaboration. We have been selected to cover a broad range of skills – from emergency medicine and infectious disease experts through to paramedics and laboratory staff. We sit in tribal groups, but a slow osmosis begins.

We quickly acclimatise to the regimentation of army life with NAAFI meals and group marches between training centres. The soldiers are welcoming and friendly to this strange invasion from clinicians. Our instructors put us to shame with their smart uniforms and impeccable manners. This is the only training day that I have been on where every session starts and ends precisely on time: I might ask them to run my life for me.

The first day explodes with questions about what is happening in Sierra Leone. The country is overtaking Liberia as the hotspot for Ebola, and the news is generally grim. This has become a complex emergency with social, economic, political, humanitarian and security dimensions. Health services are collapsing, mortality rates from common diseases such as malaria and dysentery are rising rapidly – a double whammy in a country under siege. Vaccination rates are falling, creating a legacy of childhood illness and death for the future.

MoD staff give us the background for the international efforts to contain the epidemic – Operation Gritrock (who came up with that name?). Six Ebola Treatment Centres are being built up by the British Army, though only one has managed to open so far, and that one is being set up slowly and carefully. We will be the first teams to run the next three ETCs to open.

Army medics brief us about the latest epidemiology and Porton Down doctors share their wisdom about the virus. Bats are the suspected source of this zoonotic disease, a direct source of food for subsistence farmers and an indirect agent to infect bushbuck and other forest animals which then contaminate human hunters.

Bats have a remarkable capacity to host numerous viruses such as MERS, SARS and Ebola, without experiencing any harm. They are the only mammals capable of sustained flight and to do so can generate an enormous step up in their metabolic rate that raises their core temperature to 38 degrees - a natural fever state. This may have led to genetic and immunological mechanisms that protect them from the inflammation reaction to viral exposure that causes illness in other mammals.

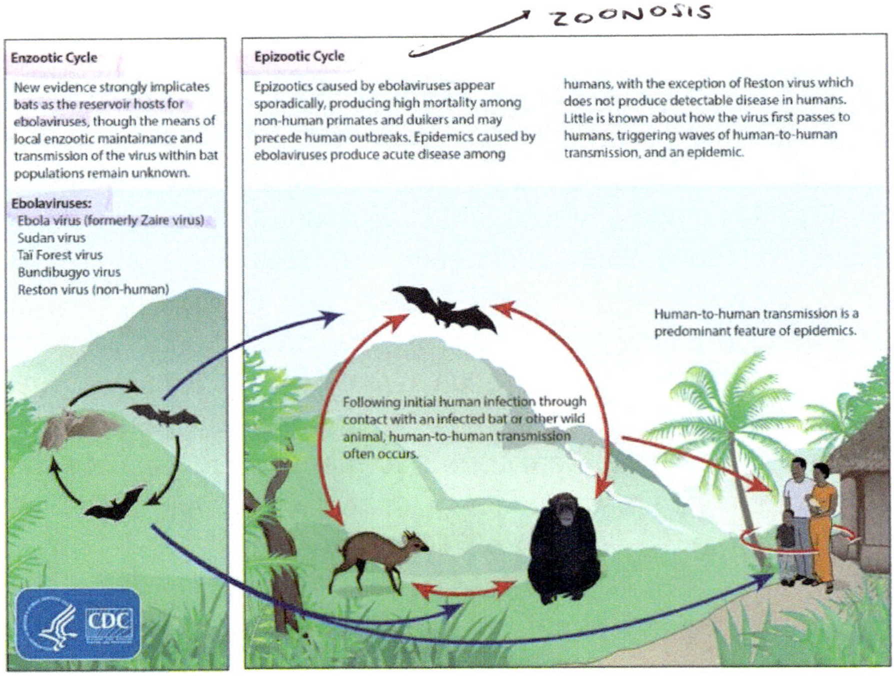

We debate recommendations for treatment for Ebola A key issue is whether we can use IV fluids – MSF have decided not to - in view of the risk of contamination of health care workers with blood. This seems a tough call to make, and potentially turns the treatment centres into palliative care centres.

A crash course in Creo to help us communicate with patients. However, all our minds are focused on the imminent training with Personal Protection Equipment (PPE) and the high fidelity training for high risk settings – three days of repetitive drills that will save our lives.

Monday, 17 November 2014
Do They Know it's Christmas Time?

Today's news headlines announce the manic success of the Band-Aid re-release of Do They Know it's Christmas. The Ebola crisis has hit home with the UK public and there is a heartfelt response to the suffering that has been reported on the television news. Paradoxically it's not money that is the priority at the moment. The UK government has committed serious funding to build and staff the six Ebola Treatment Centres in Sierra Leone. The rate limiting step is the building and the staffing of them.

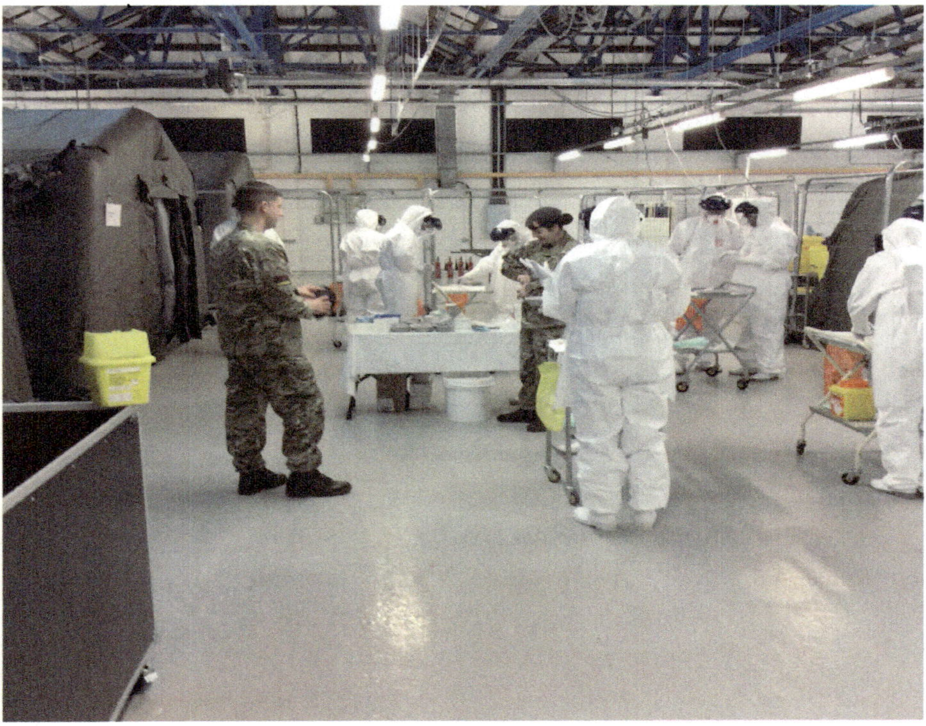

The buildings are proceeding apace with the army working furiously to complete the Centres in very difficult and often hard to reach locations. When these are ready we need to get the boots on the ground - white, rubber theatre boots in this case - and that's us.

The drills and skills training proceeds relentlessly. After five days of training we are getting impatient to get out there and help. However there is a very large cloud of fear hanging over this endeavour - that one of us gets infected - and the army and the UK government are making extra sure that this does not happen. No corners are cut and the training is ultra-rigorous.

I have now been assigned to my NGO - Medicines du Monde or Doctors of the World - a French NGO with the programme being run by the Spanish arm. I will be helping to set up the new centre in Moyamba - a 6 hour drive from the capital Freetown. My role will involve working with health services, other NGOs and local communities to make sure it works safely and effectively. The Ebola Centre is being built by the Royal Engineers with the local community, and it is planned to open on the 15th December. While the building ground is well-prepared, much work will be required between now and then to prepare the clinical ground. Imagine building, staffing and running a fully functioning district hospital in under a month.

The Ebola Centre will be staffed by the Norwegian doctors and nurses being trained with me in York. They have threatened to teach me Norwegian, but I am remarkably resistant when it comes to new languages. I have been asked to head out to Madrid as soon as my NGO can find a flight, and then straight on to Freetown. My life is moving at an increasingly fast pace, and departure is looming. Crikey.

The Ebola response is a truly international collaboration. The UK government is funding an independent emergency response team to recruit doctors and nurses for five different European NGOs. For me this involves a Spanish-led programme of a French NGO with UK funding and Norwegian clinical staff. My usual African health work involves me and an overnight bag, so this is a very different experience - a league of nations with cautious and complex decision making.

So I am heading home. Demob happy and a little bit institutionalised by army food and barracks life. My kit bag remains packed and ready for Africa.

Thursday, 20 November 2014
Waiting for a Jet Plane

Will Pooley, the nurse who 'caught' Ebola, was on the news last night bemoaning the slow response from the international community. Meanwhile we are still in Yorkshire impatient to get out and help. As this is a governmental response every i has to be dotted and every t crossed. The risk management approach is understandable, but now I just want to get on a plane to Freetown. My usual international health trips involve packing a hand luggage bag and away I go, so the slow and tortuous decision making is frustrating.

The Madrid office of Doctors of the World (Medicos del Mundo) want me to call and see them for a briefing, contract signing and another medical. I have already had a medical from DfID last week. After 50 years of successfully avoiding the clutches of the medical profession I have been caught. My systolic BP is 150 (taken in a rather intimidating war-zone field hospital tent - I hope this is passing). My potassium was 5.4 (haemolysis rather than Addisons disease I suspect), and my cholesterol was a little raised (full fry ups for army breakfasts). Otherwise I seemed to have passed for Ebola combat. However my NGO wants another test, so I will get back to my revision to pass again.

Getting on a plane is harder than it appears and flights to Freetown are getting scarce. Ryanair and Jet2 don't fly to this destination, and many airlines have stopped their normal schedules for fear of infection. Meanwhile, the entire international aid community is trying to get out to Sierra Leone. It's the opposite of the last helicopter out of Hanoi - I want the first one into Freetown. I will check the trains.

I am now getting ‘sitreps’ a catchy shortening for situational reports from the field. There really is a fog of war when it comes to international emergencies, just as there is with conflict, and the ripples of communication from the ground back to the UK become fainter with distance. The sitreps are a big help in finding out what is going on in Moyamba and the progress with the building of the Ebola Centre. Transmission of Ebola in Sierra Leone is described as intense and widespread, with over 500 cases notified in the last week. The proportion of patients isolated remains the lowest of all the West African countries, only 13%, this is due to lack of Ebola Treatment Centre and community centre facilities. 132 health care workers in Sierra Leone have been infected, with over 100 dying from the disease. The opening of the Moyamba Ebola Centre is still on track for the 15th December, so we have under 4 weeks to set up a fully functioning hospital, with lab facilities, essential drugs, 24/7 clinical rotas and clinical protocols. It feels like a big task ahead, and it's hard to solve problems from 3000 miles away.

Saturday, 22 November 2014
D-Day

A phone call from Doctors of the World and 30 minutes later I am on my way to the airport, to Madrid and my first meeting with Medicos del Mundo - the coordinating centre for my NGO. MDM was set up in 1980 by one of the founders of MSF - a splinter group with a focus on the community and political aspects of international aid. MSF are the Microsoft of aid organisations - big and powerful. MDM feels small and nimble in comparison and I am impressed by the cheerful can-do attitude of the team in the Madrid office. I meet seasoned international aid workers who reel off their tours of duty like US marines. Angola, Mozambique, Haiti, Sudan, DRC.

We sit in the cafe outside the head office in the pale winter Madrid sunshine and share concerns about the task ahead. Like mountaineers inspecting an insurmountable peak, uncertain of the best approaches to try. The time is rapidly approaching to don our protective climbing equipment and take the first tentative steps. We compare the different approaches from the UK and Spanish government. The UK has committed over £200 million, including the funding of the MDM centre. The Spanish government, they bemoan, has committed less than £20 million, and most of this is on facilities in Spain rather than Sierra Leone. After the nurse caring for an Ebola patient in Madrid became infected there is national fear of contagion, and the priority has been the home front rather than the front line.

I am spared a second medical. My DfID exam suffices, so I don't have to worry about deep breathing to control my systolic blood pressure. However, I have a psychiatric examination still to pass.

Ricardo is the seasoned MDM psychiatrist and gently probes me about how I will deal with difficult situations, isolation, ethical challenges. I feel I've had them all in my past experience, but as with my physical exam am still nervous about being found out for my latent cancer-ridden, neurotic, psychopathic traits. He is worried about the psychological effects of the suffering we will encounter, and the tendency for doctors to get frustrated and angry about not being able to do more in low resource settings and I sympathise. A pause for dramatic effect at the end of my session on the couch and I get the all clear. Do I get a certificate?

On a more mundane health matter it's time to commence my antimalarials. I always start off well with my antimalarials, usually for the first day, and then its downhill from there. However, with such government attention on this trip I vow to be more compliant. And here's the rub - I am more likely to die from malaria than Ebola in Sierra Leone. 5000 people have died from Ebola, but twice that number of children die every week from malaria in Africa. However, it's not contagious so the medicopolitcal imperative is far less than a scary, exotic viral haemorrhagic fever. There is a great cartoon of Africa in a hospital bed crying "My people is dying. Help! Help!" while the World sleeps oblivious in the visitor's chair. Next Africa cries "Epidemic can reach Western countries" and Europe awakes startled and worried.

This morning I am back to Heathrow to join my 30 NHS companions for one of the few remaining flights into Freetown. Media interest is apparently high and we have been briefed about the correct answers (these don't include 'I'm shit scared' or 'We have no idea what we are doing'). One extra complication for me is that my wallet fell out of my pocket on the Madrid flight (idiot! fool! stupido!) so I have no money, no plastic. I ring Mark my roomie from the army barracks to nervously ask if he could bring some cash for me. I feel like a living scam email - the Ebola crisis an elaborate sting for personal enrichment. Mark kindly agrees and I promise to pay him back (well......). So off to Africa for 6 weeks with £200 and no bank cards. I rationalise that it's not going to be a shopping spree.

All my electronic devices charged up in preparation for Freetown and the possibility that the city's entire electrical supply is being drained by the Apple products of the international aid community. And the greatest of all fears - no Wi-Fi.......

Sunday, 23 November 2014
Arrival in Freetown

We are seen off from Heathrow by a media scrum. The public support is amazing, though we have done nothing to deserve it yet. Flights to Freetown have dried up unsurprisingly - no Ryanair options to choose from, perhaps a good thing to reduce international spread. However, it does create a major rate limiting step in getting aid staff into the field. Our Air Moroc flight stops off in Casablanca where the tourists and business travellers leave us and we embark on a plane packed with international aid staff. MSF, CAFOD, OXFAM, Save the Children, Goal, Emergency, Doctors of the World. It feels as though we are all off to some emergency disaster annual convention.

The fever checks and hand washing begin before we even enter the customs building at Freetown airport. Then a chaotic scramble for bus seats down to the sea and a wait for a ferry that at 4am seems interminable. A snatched sleep and then we are straight to work at the MDM office in Freetown.

Three things you notice from the very first moment you arrive in Sierra Leone that illustrates the siege the country is under. First, are the security checkpoints on the road and on entry to every building where the guards are armed laser thermometers in place of guns. Everyone is stopped and their temperature checked - any sign of a fever and you don't get through. Second, are the giant vats of chlorinated water at every entrance and exit. This is the right place for obsessive compulsives - washing our hands over and over again. Third, and most unsettling is the lack of physical contact. No one touches each other, instead we mime virtual embraces and high fives. Human contact is such a fundamental part of how we demonstrate our friendship and our love, so its removal creates a strange emotional loss. Imagine a society without touch.

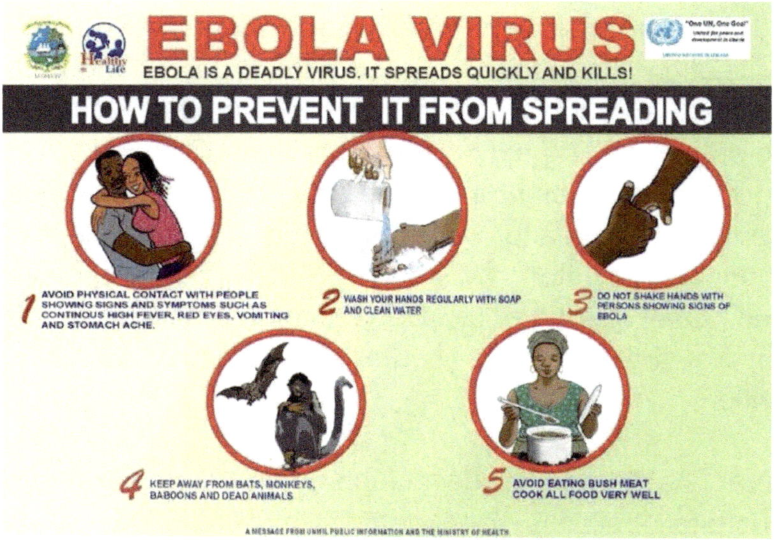

We join a team of four colleagues from Madrid and together we have to get the Ebola Centre safe and operational in 3 weeks. Top priorities that we are going to have to tackle are:

1. The Royal Engineers want an urgent meeting to make sure they have built the right facilities. DfID are offering to fly three of us out to Moyamba to do this in one of the three helicopters on HMS Argos, moored in the harbour off Freetown. I selflessly volunteer.
2. We have to get a lab ready quickly, otherwise we will not be able to diagnose Ebola cases, and the treatment centre will end up full of patients with malaria, pneumonia etc, risking cross infection with those patients who do have Ebola. The US military have offered a mobile PCR lab, but we need to agree numbers of lab staff to run it and where it can be located.
3. We need to agree the supply of the medical equipment necessary to run the centre. DfID procurement advisors tell us that this will be 300m3 - this is six sea containers worth of kit and we will need to find out where to store it and how to find the supplies we need when we need them.
4. We need to employ local staff - nurses, health care assistants, cooks, cleaners, drivers. This will involve numerous interviews and then appropriate training. We will start this tomorrow.
5. We need a base camp near the centre to house all the national and international staff. The Norwegian military are building this, but work has been delayed as we agree appropriate non-Ebola medevac arrangements.
6. We need to work up clinical rotas for the doctors and nurses without much idea about how many we will need to cover 24/7 care in the 'red zone'.

Too much to do, too little time.

Tuesday, 25 November 2014
Faster, Faster...

There is a continuing tension about the speed of opening of the Ebola Centres and the safety of staff working in them. The UK government has funded six 100 bed centres. Six hundred beds is probably a fraction of what is needed, but still only one is open (Kerrytown) and less than 10 beds in this centre are being used - with patients being turned away. Last week, a Cuban doctor from the Kerrytown centre was evacuated to Geneva having had a nosocomial (hospital acquired) Ebola infection. The fear of another case paralyses the rapid increase in capacity that is needed to treat all the patients with Ebola out in the community, and so the epidemic continues to spread.

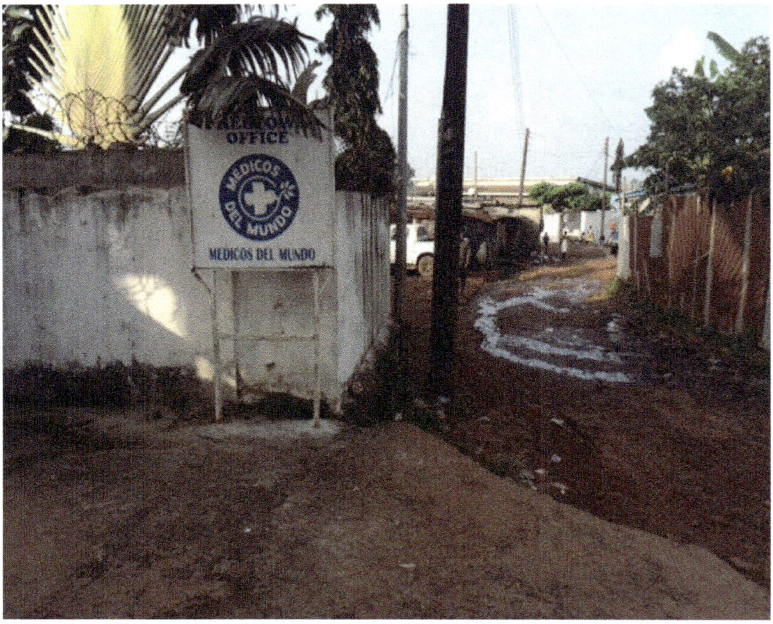

I meet one of the senior Ministry of Health doctors who bemoans the seemingly snails pace of the Centres. In neighbouring Liberia the US military has built 17 centres and these are all apparently operational. Faster, faster - our people are dying. Yet caution dominates the agenda. We need a better understanding of why health care workers are getting contaminated - more root cause analysis of contributory factors so that the lessons can be learnt quickly and steps taken to improve safety of care. At the moment risk aversion is creating a lag to an effective Ebola response.

RHETORICAL QUESTIONS - WHAT ARE THESE

One of the central issues related to risk is how interventional we should be with patients. Should we be using IV fluids? Central lines? Inotropes? Doctors inevitably want to do as much as they can, to be as interventional as they are trained, but in this situation a more conservative approach to care may be warranted. This is a tricky moral maze to tread.

Meanwhile, the urgency in setting up our own centre continues. I meet with Susan Elden who is a DfID health advisor, and one of my previous public health trainees who I worked with in Swaziland. She shares the same frustration about speed of progress and describes the mud-wading she has to go through in coordinating so many different national and international partners. It feels quite liberating to be working on the ground, away from the political games that partners are playing with this toxic football.

Our small team is working well, a good chemistry and formidable commitment. We start shortlisting our first group of staff for training - 30 this week, then 30 more the next week and up to 90 for the opening. Tomorrow we head to Moyamba for our first visit to meet the Royal Engineers and the local community.

Wednesday, 26 November 2014
Ebola junction - first glimpse

A long and dusty journey over red African roads to Moyamba and our first sight of the final stages of the building of our Ebola Centre. Staff Sergeant Adam proudly shows us around, his team of Royal Engineers having worked every hour for four weeks to build a fully functioning mini-hospital. They had returned from Afghanistan only to be sent straight out to help this new war. Taliban. Ebola. It's all the same really.

We take a patient journey, through the triage and on to the suspected Ebola ward, then the probable Ebola ward until they get to the confirmed Ebola ward. This is the high risk red zone which will be the most dangerous part of the Centre. Bore holes, giant water containers and huge chlorine vats will provide our life blood of disinfection. Decontamination areas and fearsome incinerators will dispose of our very toxic waste. Air conditioned laboratory and pharmacy. Hanger size dining rooms and storage spaces.

It's a remarkable facility - £1.5 million worth, cut out of dense African jungle. Even at the height of the epidemic it is hard not to stop thinking about how it can be used when this is all over. However this remains a long way away, and in the meantime we have to turn this building site into an ultra-sterile hospital within three weeks. The size of the challenge is daunting.

Another case of an infected health care worker from an Ebola Centre, the second expatriate evacuated within a week. There is a mounting sense of panic and fear. There is a real urgency to understand what the root causes are for these serious safety failures. In medicine we make lots of comparisons with the airline industry in our quest to improve safety. The big difference with airlines however, is that if something goes wrong on a plane, it is the pilot who dies first as it crashes into a mountainside. In healthcare, it is the patient that dies when a serious error occurs - never the doctor. Until now. Here in Sierra Leone it is the health care workers who are dying when mistakes are made and the urgency to improve safety is suddenly much more urgent.

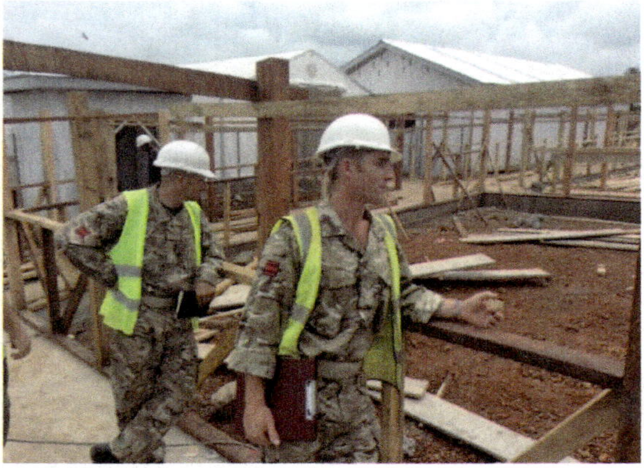

We meet the Norwegian military team who are building the base camp for the international staff. One big decision, taken by government mandarins in Oslo, is that no Sierra Leonians will be allowed into the camp. We protest strongly at this new Ebola apartheid, which makes little scientific sense and transmits a nasty undertone to the national staff we will be recruiting, who will be taking the same risks as us. However this is a political decision infused by fear. No risk will be taken with international staff. Even the 20 Norwegian base camp workers will have separate ablution facilities to their Norwegian clinical colleagues to minimise any potential risk.

Moyamba is a sleepy African backwater, and accommodation for our MDM team turns out to be limited. The Norwegians have tents only for themselves. The Royal Engineers kindly offer shelter in a disused stadium that has been their home for the last 6 weeks. They introduce us to the magic of British Army self-heating rations and like wide-eyed kids in a sweet shop we are spoilt for choices that include chicken tikka, pasta Bolognese, chilli con carne. The addition of water and a few minutes later we are scooping mouthfuls of disappointing and indistinguishable food from plastic bags, but we are hungry and grateful.

They also offer to share their trickle of Wi-Fi and we scramble for precious internet and emails, feeling out of place among all the uniformed soldiers with their 'Sniper' T shirts and camouflage fatigues.

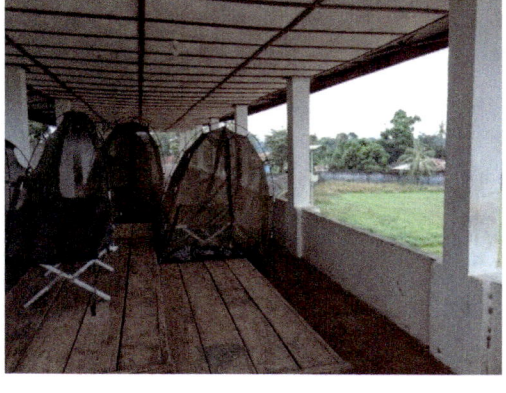

Sleeping quarters adjoin the makeshift kitchen and common room. Rows of camp beds stretch into the dark corners where soldiers pass the empty evening illuminated by their mobile phones and tablets. We are offered a camp bed amongst the rows but are not quite ready for such close communal living with the young squaddies. We grab a mosquito net and head up the stairs to the top tier of the grandstand overlooking a sad, overgrown football pitch, bedding down with the company of swarms of mosquitoes. We had assumed our Sierra Leonian drivers would join us, but at the last minute I am gently taken aside and informed that this is not allowed. No nationals allowed. That's the rules. It takes me back to travelling in South Africa during the dark apartheid days.

Thursday, 27 November 2014
Care in the Community

A hot, noisy night full of mosquitoes but empty of sleep. Today is a chance to get linked in to the local community and make sure that the Ebola Centre does not become a white (African) elephant, shunned when it opens, nor an isolated island in the existing district health system stream. I attend the regular morning Command and Control meeting, run as the name suggests by the Sierra Leonean army. National politics overtook the running of the national Ebola response in early November when the President essentially fired the Ministry of Health and asked the Royal Sierra Leonean army to take over. Not surprisingly there is a tension between the two approaches – the army full of tactics and the Ministry of Health full of strategy.

The Command and Control meeting is run in full military style with barked orders and updates. The officer running the meeting informs us that if any suspected Ebola patient tries to get too close at a checkpoint then the usual army terms of engagement will be followed. It brings up images of a whole new form of delayed-detonation suicide attacks at security checkpoints.

Then to a community briefing of local stakeholders from the Royal Engineers and an opportunity to meet the local Paramount Chief. Moyamba is one of 14 chiefdoms in the district and paradoxically, as the location of the Ebola Treatment Centre, appears to have been the least affected. Chief Gulama, the rather suave and snappily dressed community leader ascribes their local success to robust checkpoints that have kept the Ebola patients from other chiefdoms at bay. I ask him if he is worried about the sudden influx of Ebola patients to this town when the Centre opens its doors, but he seems prouder of the achievements of its location here than any threat to his Ebola defences.

Everyone is impatient. They need the centre to open now, and while the 15th December seems scarily close to me, it is an age away for the community who have set up their own holding centre to isolate patients in the absence of any more appropriate clinical facilities. I will have to take a look at this holding centre when I get the chance – sounds a bit like a concentration camp.

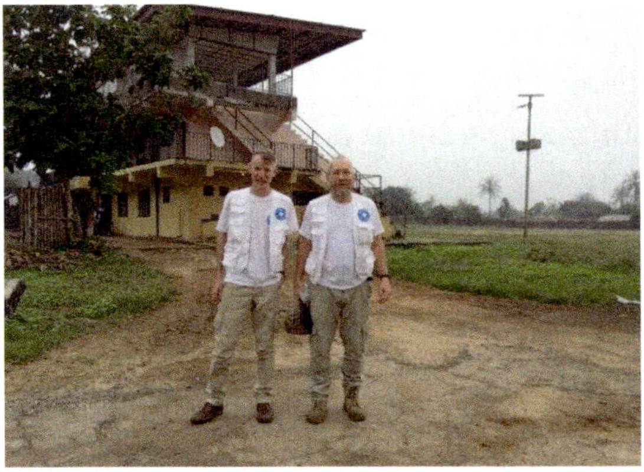

USAID come down from Freetown to investigate how their recent offer of a fully staffed PCR lab will fit into the Ebola Centre plans. Within a few minutes of their arrival it becomes clear that it won't. The beautifully constructed Ebola Centre laboratory is not the space they are looking for – in typical American fashion their intention is to bring a fully functioning stand-alone lab and helicopter it in (complete with 12 staff). The Royal Engineers Staff Sergeant smiles and gently shakes his head. I am waiting for him to say that it is possible, but it is going to cost us. There does not appear to be enough space on this tightly designed floorplan and the USAID folk head back to Freetown to discuss with their Department of Defence. Meanwhile we need to get a plan B.

We shortlist our first 20 local nurses and arrange for WHO training to start tomorrow. In addition we need an army of 'hygienists' who can help decontaminate the wards. This sweet-sounding title essentially involves clearing up all the extremely toxic blood, vomit and diarrhea from the Ebola patients, so it's not going to be a hugely enticing job description. However, we will need people with intelligence, care and precision to undertake this most dangerous of roles. Fortunately for us (though less fortunately for the education of an entire generation of school children) all the schools have been closed in an effort to reduce person-to-person spread. This provides a crucial pool of unemployed school teachers who are keen for work and we can be confident will pass the intensive training.

On the way out of the Ebola Centre building site I ask the local contractor for his observations about the epidemic. He tells me that one unintended consequence is that nobody is having sex anymore, and infidelity has disappeared. A biblical plague indeed.

Friday, 28 November 2014
Q: Why is this Ebola out break so bad? A: We were late

Back to the big city for our final preparation before we set up base in Moyamba for good. We need somewhere to stay on our return and have asked the Norwegians if we can camp with them while they build the base camp. They have erected large eight-person tents, but only sufficient room for their forward party, and they still need to build basic facilities for the new guests. We have left them hammering and sawing in the fine Scandinavian Ikea style.

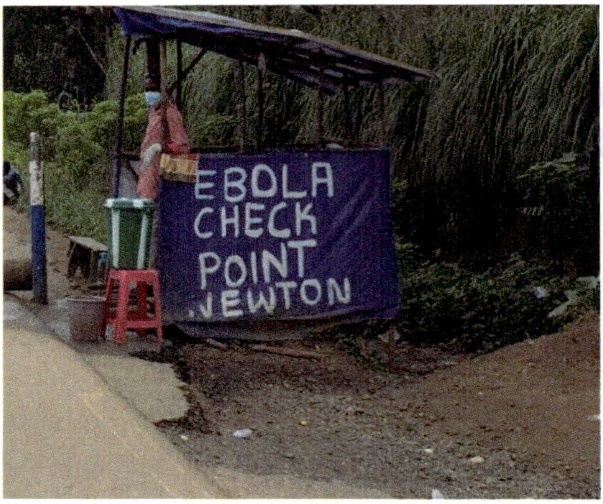

The latest UN Emergency Ebola Response 'sitrep' for Sierra Leone is out. 6535 cases and 1367 deaths. I don't understand why the mortality is so low - some recording bias or case ascertainment I suspect. In health care workers the numbers are 136 and 105 - 77% mortality, which is much more in keeping with what we would expect, and the case ascertainment and reporting will be more accurate. Only 53% of Ebola cases are being isolated, and 60% having safe burials within 24 hours; so much work to do. The target for Ebola Treatment beds is 1500 with only 500 in operation.

The country now needs 200,000 Personal Protection Equipment suits every month to cope with clinical demand. For us the debate rages over goggles or visors. We have all been trained with visors and have been told that the goggles are terrible to wear - fogging up in the heat within minutes and dangerously reducing vision. However MSF are entrenched in their view that hoods and goggles are the safest and we appear to have stepped unwittingly into a religious crusade with dogma and evangelicalism in place of reason and dialogue. I email Professor Nigel Silman at Porton Down who helped develop our PPE and he reassures me that there is no evidence that either method is safer. We will keep the visor faith for now.

A new arrival in the office today with Julio, our watsan (water and sanitation) expert. He will take the lead for the safe decontamination of any potential sources of infection leaving the red zone. New rules in the MDM office are quickly established to reinforce that hygiene begins at home. He tells us we need separate water bottles to pour our water, which seems a particularly paranoid approach - drinking out of the same bottle I understand, but having to write our names on each water bottle for pouring? He views the world through a particular microbe-covered lens, but that is exactly the sort of obsessional perspective we need at the moment. Without any sense of irony he demonstrates the safest method to take and light a cigarette to minimise contact and protect health. We go over the Ebola Centre plans to identify potential breaches in the armour, and list changes that may be required.

We gatecrash the WHO Ebola briefing which seems preoccupied with the design of a data collection form for a national audit. One and half hours into a very slow meeting I text Chris who is sitting opposite with a request to kill me quickly. The highlight is a drop-in visit from Mike Ryan who is the director of the WHO's alert and response operations and has been involved in an impressive 19 out of the last 20 Ebola epidemics. I ask him why this one is so bad. The answer is simple - we were late. He describes how viruses like influenza spread in waves affecting everybody, whereas Ebola spreads in a more sinister fashion, travelling undetected along channels until it finds a weak point, a burial or a poorly run health centre, and then it explodes. Health care workers are the mine canaries - their deaths providing the critical warning for an epidemic.

Mike is concerned about some of the Ebola Centres becoming 'amplification' centres - where misdiagnosed cases mix with Ebola patients and then go home to carry on transmission. Also, that we need to balance the approach to looking after patients across the spectrum of community centres and holding units and not just on Ebola Treatment Centres - if we get it wrong upstream we will end up seeing patients at death's door and having to undertake high risk interventional procedures that are risky to the clinicians and mostly futile for the patient. If we get it right then we will be able to manage them simply and safely. I will have to go and explore the community centres and holding centres, though I am nervous about exposure in these low-protection areas, so will have to be cautious. Being in the red zone, fully kitted out and fully trained is probably the safest place to be in this epidemic. It is the less rigorously controlled community settings where danger lurks.

The informal discussions after the meeting are the most useful and we get some invaluable tips for what we will need - which guidelines to use, mentoring for the staff when we open, reassurance about the clinical side ('It's actually pretty boring from a medical perspective - just one disease'). Also insight into Kerrytown over which clouds appear to have gathered. One lesson from this ETC is that they opened their doors to everyone on the first day and were quickly overrun. We need to adopt a measured approach and manage community expectations as we take our first tentative steps.

Saturday, 29 November 2014
The Apartheid of Ebola

There is a strange separateness in the country, a new apartheid of Ebola. It manifests itself at an individual level in the enforced physical separateness of individuals, but also an apartheid between the new wave of international visiting aid workers and the Sierra Leonians, or nationals as they are referred to in a rather de-personalised manner. International staff are under strict orders to minimise contact with nationals. So public transport is forbidden, even taxi rides. I'm used to the white people in African countries driving around in large 4x4s, but here it is an absolute separation in transport. International staff are told to stay in their compounds - no early evening walks into town or mingling in shops or restaurants. They are prisoners in the country they have come to liberate.

Everyone is habituated into the endless routines of chlorine hand washing, but for the international staff personal hygiene has reached Howard Hughes levels of obsession with bottles of alcohol gel carried like silver crosses to ward away this invisible vampire. There is little evidence that Ebola hangs around on surfaces for long - probably just a few hours. But this uncertainty is enough to sow a seed of fear that rapidly consumes your daily routine, and I find myself, against my rational

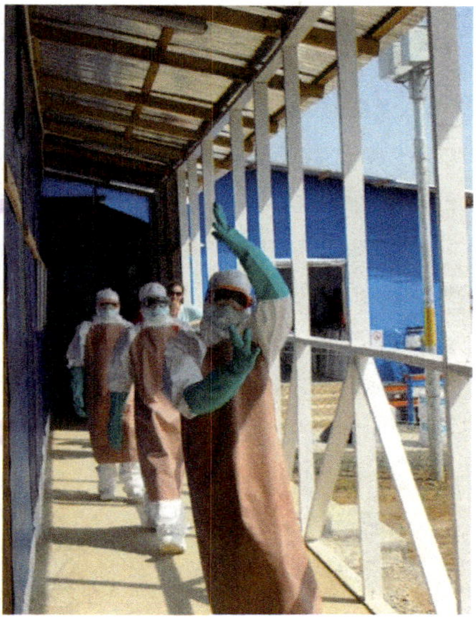

nature, reflexively avoiding unknown foreign surfaces, towels. Even money becomes a potential vehicle for transmission in my over-heated mind.

Today I have my first visit to an Ebola Centre. Rachel Cummings the Health Advisor from Save the Children gives us an expert guided tour and we see care in full action. It's an impressive show, and she emphasises that it is a full hospital in all but name. They have had a stormy time over the last few days, having been open nearly a month and yet having only 25 patients through their doors. It's an impossible position for them - with Cuban clinicians, UK management, WHO oversight and DfID funding. The flashbulbs of the UK media are on them, all impatient for news about how they have single handedly eliminated Ebola. I am glad we are away from the media spotlight.

There is so much for us to learn from their first few weeks as we tour and observe. My takeaway list includes

1) Start with confirmed cases only - otherwise we will be swamped with demand
2) Start slowly and work up to full capacity while we test our clinical processes and safety
3) Cold drinking water for staff. We watched them being decontaminated and undressed - soaked with sweat and exhausted after less than an hour in the red zone
4) Prepare everything - IV packs, bloods, drugs etc before we enter the red zone - reduce risk of needlesticks etc. while in PPE
5) Clocks on every wall to keep a close track of time - like divers under water

6) We need to develop methods of communication between the red and green zones - they use walkie talkies, but not ideal.
7) Lots of photos of ward layouts to we can replicate the templates in Moyamba
8) Protocols for children - especially where the mother dies under care. Rachel describes a recent case where the mother was admitted late stage and died, but her infant son by some miracle was negative.

Now we have a model that we can work towards and we take our photographs back to base to plan.

EXAMPLES OF LIC'S
> POOR PUBLIC
HEALTH.

Monday, 1 December 2014
Epidemics: Consequences of Poor Public Health

Here's an interesting discovery. In 2012 there was a major cholera epidemic in West Africa. Three countries were mainly affected - Sierra Leone, Liberia and Guinea. Two years later in 2014 these same three countries are at the centre of the Ebola epidemic. This is not random bad luck. The root causes of these infectious epidemics lies in poor basic public health: a lack of clean water; the absence of a proper sewage system. Health systems that have become frail and fragile whether through the consequence of civil war or benign neglect and underinvestment.

The UK government is investing £230 million to help contain the Ebola epidemic in Sierra Leone. This is being matched with donations from other international donors. So half a billion pounds will be burnt in this particular fire, and this is just a fraction of what the cost of the Ebola epidemic will be to the country through economic stagnation and health services collapse.

The cholera epidemic was undoubtedly a mine canary for Ebola - a serious early warning of this subsequent critical event. Half a billion pounds invested in public health development in 2014, providing clear water and effective sanitation, would have been a better investment in the long term health of the country than expensive Ebola Treatment Centres that, when this is over, will be consumed by the African bush as quickly as they were built. Hindsight bias can be a lazy informant, but it's hard not to walk through sliding doors into different possible worlds. Just as we undertake a serious incidence investigation into the root causes of errors that lead to a patient's death in hospital, we must look back at the root causes of the Ebola epidemic and learn lessons. But this is for the future - there are more pressing matters to deal with.

Susan Elden from DfID invites us to the regular 8pm briefing at the ISAT compound, the base for the UK military attachment. We enter late to the ops room packed full of fatigue-clad army officers, standing in rows around a large table upon which a giant map of the country is pinned down. Crisp military replies to urgent questions provide the latest update for the emergency. The President has been visiting sites with DfID and urging his chiefs to pick up the pace in surveillance and detection. Progress from the Royal Engineers in completing the 5 remaining sites is good. There is a communication problem with the UK media which is focusing entirely on Kerrytown - one story suggesting that the £230 million has just been for this Ebola Centre. One of the helicopters is out of service for a day while its engine is repaired.

It is a war room in everything but name. Under the surface of the calm military precision there is a sense that political pressures are being brought to bear. This is an election year in the UK - and the government's Ebola response must be seen to be an international success - the UK saving the world once again. This political expediency bears no relation to the reality of the challenges we face on the ground, of building and opening hospitals at speed in remote locations and making absolutely sure none of our NHS staff are put at risk.

The US Department of Defence look as though they are backtracking on our much needed lab. The meeting provides a good opportunity to nobble the senior DfID advisors and ask for political help and the search for alternative donors.

Monday, 1 December 2014
Laka: An Interventional Approach

The week slips seamlessly into the weekend. No one rests in the Ebola response teams. We visit our second Ebola Centre. This time in Laka, nearer to Freetown than Kerrytown, run by an Italian NGO called Emergency (great name). Emergency have a small Ebola Centre but will be moving next door to a brand new, UK funded Ebola Treatment Centre, just like ours at Moyamba, opening the day before we do in Moyamba. They have been working in Freetown for 13 years and been active in treating Ebola patients since the start of the epidemic, opening a standalone unit in September. This is a Heath Robinson model compared to the Royal Engineers beautiful design, but it works well. I am reunited for a brief time with some of my colleagues from training in York who look as though they have been managing Ebola for years - seasoned professionals. I watch them in admiration as they captain this fleet of tented ships.

Emergency are unashamedly interventional. There is a spectrum of debate about Ebola Centres that ranges from viewing them as a public health intervention - essentially to isolate patients and to provide conservative management, reducing risk to staff, through to Emergency who think that there should not be double standards. Survival in the West is 70%, yet only 30% in Africa, and this inequality should be unacceptable. So they intervene as doctors like to do so much - every patient gets a catheter, and IV line, a central line, even ventilation. I ask about survival, and am told it is 30-40%, and wonder if their approach is worth it. I am sympathetic to their noble philosophy. If I got Ebola, it would be a good place to come to. However, the equality they strive to provide only exists in this tiny pocket of Africa, and while it would be great to offer everyone kidney transplants and expensive new drugs, it is not sustainable in a low resource setting. The benefit this approach offers is probably marginal compared to providing basic health care: immunisations, maternal health, essential drugs and universal access to primary care.

The difference between Kerrytown and Laka is noteworthy. Kerrytown started from scratch in a bespoke, but untested Ebola Treatment Centre. They were plunged into the deep end, without any opportunity to learn to swim. Their first month of operation has involved an enormous challenge of adapting their facility to the needs and demands of their patients. Laka in contrast grew organically to meet the growing needs of patients in their community. They were well established and able to test and evolve in true quality improvement fashion. Hundreds of small changes over time to develop the model that works for them. It's a classic example of top down versus organic, bottom up approaches to change. However, in this case the urgency of the epidemic and the lack of suitable Laka-like sites provided little option but to adopt an imposed response.

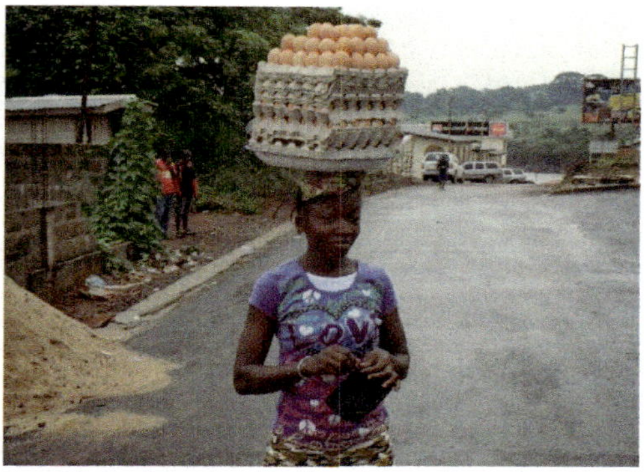

I manage for the first time to shake off my protective bubble and take a walk through the crowded back streets of Freetown. Tin music blares loudly from the tin huts that line the earthen roads. Women sway with impossible loads balanced effortlessly on their heads. Children dance around my legs. Chickens and goats scatter in my path. Heat, noise, smells, sights, laughter.

I see a young women with dozens of eggs balanced precariously on her head and I feel a personal metaphor for my fragile task ahead: I've got all my eggs in one ETC basket, balanced on my head.

My senses are engulfed with this joyous humanity, and with a sudden, unexpected choking, I realise my loss, my disconnection from this essence of Africa. I have become so engrossed and single-minded in my mission I have forgotten where I am. My relentless mindfulness about labs, recruitment, training, drug supply, types of protective equipment has drowned out the people's lives that this disaster response is all about.

Enough of the planning already. Time to act. To Moyamba tomorrow for handover, and then to Bo for my first experience in the red zone.

Tuesday, 2 December 2014
Behaviour Change: the Holy Grail of Health Care

One last meeting in the big city. Donal Brown, Head of the UK Ebola Task Force, kindly agrees to meet me at the very lovely ISAT compound. He leads the military and DfID response in Sierra Leone and offers an honest and thoughtful reflection of the current emergency. This is the largest and most complex disaster response programme that DfID has undertaken. He tells me how most disasters strike and then recede. Ebola in contrast just gets bigger and bigger. Most of DfID's programmes involve simple interventions such as vaccination programmes or medical support. This war on Ebola is dependent on changing people's behaviour - how they treat the dead, burials, not touching in a very tactile society. Behaviour change is the Holy Grail for most of health care, but nowhere as urgent as here.

He tells me that with Ebola the speed of the emergency is such that a day is a week, a week is a month and a month is a year. He is clearly proud of the UK's response - how the army has built 5 mini-hospitals that would normally take a year, all in 6 weeks. The Task Force has tried to take a whole system approach, not just focusing on the Ebola Centres. In particular, the command and control structure run by the UK and Sierra Leonean Military has enabled effective coordination of notifications, alerts, transport of cases and isolation. The final, but critical, link in the chain is the beds at the Ebola Centres. I push him on when we will get ahead of the infection curve and, not surprisingly, he is cautious - the first quarter of 2015 he offers with wide confidence intervals.

I bring my list of 'challenges' (problems) no lab yet (!); how are we going to deal with 300m3 of stores; we need PPE to train our new staff with; difficulties with the Norwegian base camp; organising the inauguration (optimistically). I also want to try to install CCTV to provide a simple and cheap method for monitoring staff and patient safety. He makes phone calls and solves problems. Wonderful. He rushes off with the promise to visit us.

Wednesday, 3 December 2014
The Politics, Philosophy and Economics of PPE

This is my life. I wake at dawn after a fitful sleep, unaccustomed to the heat and the noise, waking during the night with a list of problems running through my head. If I have internet, than I catch up on emails while I await a lift from my guesthouse. Then we work together in whatever office space we can find, covering the tasks in order of today's priorities, drawing smaller and smaller circles around them until they have disappeared. Meals are sporadic and always very late. Food is basic in Moyamba, though the Norwegians take pity on us and drop round a box of army rations. In Moyamba there is no running water, so I remain dusty and sweaty during the day. The Royal Engineers wash in bottled water – Cleopatra-like with Evian in place of ass's milk – but they have no room for us now. Work continues until fatigue sets in, then to bed and the cycle continues. I have nothing tangible to show for my efforts at the end of the day, just a mind map that hangs over my bed every night like a child's mobile.

So we are all chronically tired, hungry, smelly and hot. Perhaps it is not surprising that the arrival of a new influx of international staff generates some tensions. Tiredness and uncertainty in our rapidly assembled and unfamiliar team leads to disagreements about how fast we should open, how interventional our treatment should be, and always, what sort of protective equipment is best. The type of PPE, personal protective equipment, to use is the Middle East politics of Ebola. If you trained in visors you believe in visors, in goggles then you believe in goggles. A night's rest and reflection and gentle stroking and we are soon back on course.

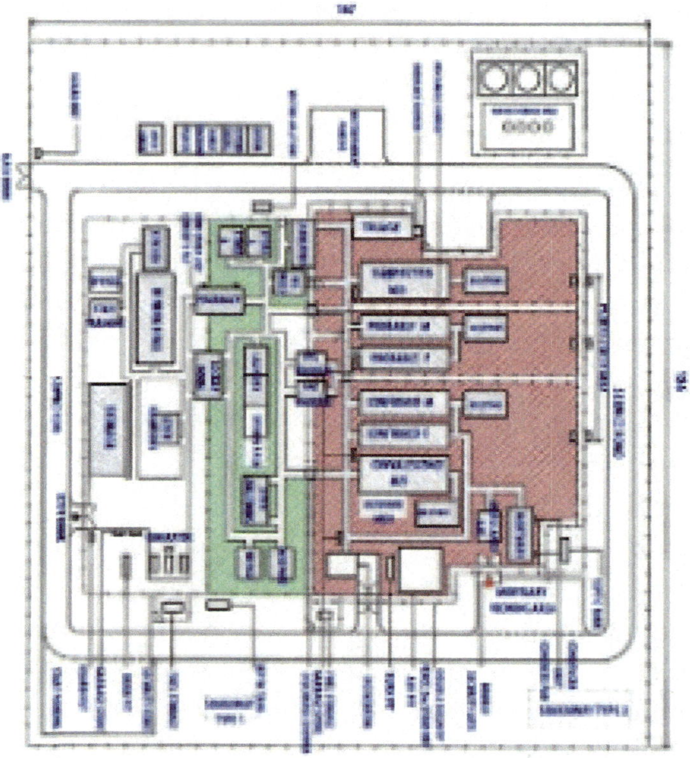

Great progress has been made since my last visit to the Ebola Centre in Moyamba. The site – 8 football pitches in size – is nearing completion, though JCB diggers still race around in a frenetic ballet. We take beneficiary occupancy from the Royal Engineers and DfID – I'm not really sure what this means, but for the first time we have fenced off buildings, and tents that we can access without hard hats and high vis jackets. We will start unloading our supplies when the World Food Programme delivers them in a couple of days. It's an unfamiliar world of logistics and facilities management and I have little to contribute.

Royal Navy helicopters make regular trips from HMS Argus, moored off Freetown, to the stadium where they unload urgent supplies. It's all very Top Gun, though the coolness factor of the pilots is let down by their Health and Safety requirement to don safety goggles and ear protectors every time they jump on and off.

Progress is happening. The Americans have been threatening to install their donated lab an hour's drive away at the junction with the main tarmac road – easier access for them perhaps, but it makes no sense for us, so we call in another offer and one day later the US embassy comes back with confirmation that they will install it where we want it at the Centre. I also manage to recruit a pharmacist. There is only one applicant – fresh out of college, but bright and eager and local, so a 3 minute interview and he has instructions to turn up on Friday ready to stock and prepare for dispensing the Centre's pharmacy.

There is one big missing piece in our Ebola jigsaw. None of us have ever seen a case of Ebola before. This is not a good situation with the blind leading the blind when we open in 2

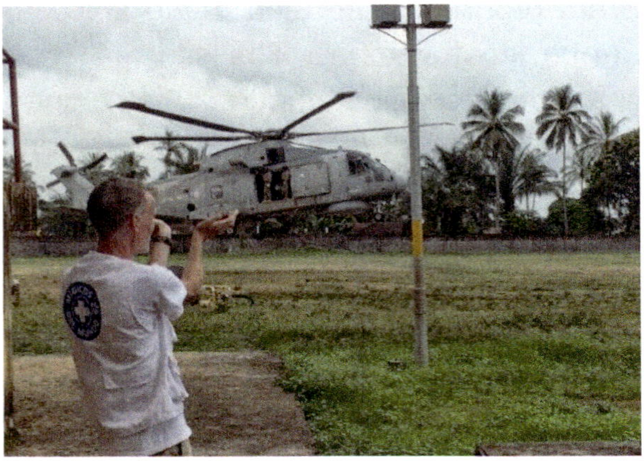

weeks' time. Getting experience is a bit of a Catch 22, and the existing Ebola Centres are too busy to offer practical experience. So Chris and I are off to Bo – a three hour drive from Moyamba, deeper into the heart of Africa to take up an offer to work on the wards at the MSF Ebola Centre in the town.

At the last minute I manage to hitch a ride on the UN helicopter. Having never been in a helicopter this gives me an unashamedly boyish thrill as it lands in the middle of the abandoned stadium where the Royal Engineers are based. The excitement is extinguished suddenly as the staff sergeant explodes with fury that the UN have landed at what is a full military forward operating base without permission. The ancient Mi-26 Soviet helicopter is surrounded by armed British soldiers and the staff sergeant screams at the pilots over the noise of the decelerating rotors that they would be entitled to shoot the helicopter down for the incursion.

The Russian pilot shrugs with Slavic indifference, a cigarette hanging out of the side of his mouth "So vat are you going to do eh, shoot us?". "There is going to be an international shitstorm" the staff sergeant mutters to me as I grab my bag and leap aboard, escaping the guilt about provoking WW3, and anticipating the "UK declares war on UN" headlines in the morning papers.

And so we go to Bo. This is one of the most experienced Ebola treatment centres, and while I am starting to feel that I have had more training in Ebola than I had for my entire medical career, I know that my ultimate test is when I enter the red zone.

Thursday, 4 December 2014
Rats for Lassa, Dogs for Rabies, Mosquitoes for Malaria, Humans for Ebola

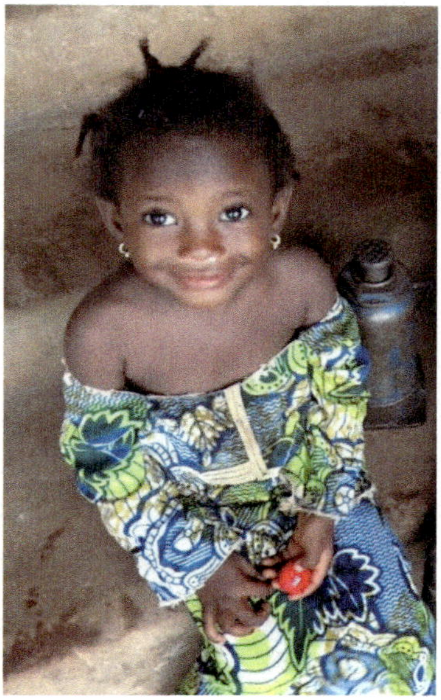

Another international health worker has been infected with Ebola, the third in the ten days since I have been here. This time an American, flown out by one of the only two planes equipped with the very expensive isolation pods - $250,000 a flight. WHO have been working on a standard approach to medevac and have agreed that all suspected cases will be sent immediately to the UK military facility co-located in Kerrytown, and then on to the most appropriate specialist medical centre. There was a problem with the Cuban medic as the American planes couldn't breach US embargo and land in Havana, so he has been taken to Geneva.

There is clearly a different price on international heads. The cases amongst Sierra Leonean health workers pass unnoticed whereas each international case sparks an anxious, rumour-driven chain of whispers. Some cases are attributed to the type of personal protective equipment - the duck-bill masks becoming soaked in sweat until they cause a sense of drowning and panic - Ebola waterboarding. Other cases appear to be linked to the high risk admission of patients through triage in Ebola centres, before they get to the sanctuary of the red zone. Some infections appear to be transmitted in the community - causal encounters or patients calling to health care workers' homes to seek help. The risks are small, but very real and the uncertainty about common cause is unsettling.

Last night, as I was walking back from town to my guest house a young boy grabbed my hand. It was an affectionate gesture, a curious child. It was the first time anyone has touched me in nearly two weeks, and my immediate response was one of warmth, discovery of a long lost sense. However, a couple of seconds later and I was racked with doubt. Who was the boy? Did his hand seem hot? I keep my hand out at a distance until I arrive home, and then I'm all Lady Macbeth with my alcohol gel and soap.

At the MSF headquarters in Bo an obstetrician tells me about the devastating impact of Ebola on maternity care. The bleeding related to this haemorrhagic disease has led to few pregnant women surviving, and almost none of the babies. Worse still is the dismantling of routine antenatal healthcare: the loss of health care staff through Ebola; the fear of expectant mothers to go near an Ebola-infested health facility; a rise in pregnancy rates in high risk mothers from unplanned and teenage pregnancies. Maternal mortality in the UK is 8.4 per 100,000 women. In Sierra Leone it has been recorded as nearly 5,000 per 100,000 and latest data suggests this has risen to 14,000 per 100,000 - almost 1 in every 7 pregnant women dying before delivery. The danger from Ebola pales in comparison.

RATS — ANIMAL CARRYING LOTS OF VIRUSES

> EBOLA
> LASSA

Bo is at the heart of another viral haemorrhagic disease: Lassa fever. Over 5,000 people die every year from this one, but its spread is mainly through rats, and it's less of a contagious risk to the world, geographically confined to this region in West Africa. So, like malaria, we can turn a blind eye to the death and suffering it causes, unless you happen to be living here. We are told to be on rat alert, keeping food and rubbish tightly sealed. Also, to be careful of the rabid dogs. Rats for Lassa, dogs for rabies, mosquitoes for malaria, humans for Ebola - I'm living in a kind of apocalyptic inter-species World War III.

Meanwhile a rather sad string of Christmas tinsel has been hung up outside the town's hotel. So the answer to Band Aid's question is: yes.

Friday, 5 December 2014
All Fevers are Ebola: Unless Proven Otherwise

The WHO likes dividing its operations into clusters and pillars. For Ebola there are 6 pillars supporting the emergency response:

1) Isolation of patients - this is the main role of our expensive Ebola Treatment Centres - more quarantine centres than treatment centres
2) Safe burials - Ebola is at its most dangerous in the final stages and after death - a clever evolutionary trick
3) Awareness raising - changing behaviours of an entire population - to notify cases, to wash hands and stop touching
4) Alert and surveillance - basic epidemiology to help inform the who, where and when of Ebola and to monitor trends.

5) Contact tracing - this is always low down for infection control in Africa (e.g. TB where it always happens in the UK, but rarely happens in Africa), but for Ebola the efforts have been ramped up
6) Health access for non-Ebola cases. It is this pillar that we delve into today.

At Bo we are being taught by MSF how to run an Ebola Centre and some of the many lessons they have learnt. MSF have had 25 of their health workers infected with Ebola - 22 national and 3 international. Most of these are dead. Today we deal with how to handle fevers in staff. There is a bit of tramline thinking when it comes to fevers and it's important not to forget the other common causes (malaria, Lassa etc). However what MSF have found is that staff are cautious about coming forward. They have seen at first hand the suffering and mostly fatal outcomes of the patients on the wards, and this is the last place they want to get sent to. So they cover up and they self-medicate, all the while increasing the risk of spread to their colleagues.

So, a proactive approach has been adopted. All staff have thermometers and do thrice daily temperatures (must remember to start doing mine). The cheap Chinese laser thermometers are not trusted, so all staff need to measure their axillary temperature before they leave home, and then on arrival at the Ebola Centre. They are only let in to the Ebola Centre when they show the reading to the security guard. Bed nets and antimalarials are provided to all staff now in order to reduce the chance of malaria and the fear that a malaria fever will bring (all fevers are Ebola until proven otherwise). Personal hygiene kits are given to everyone for use at home. The no-touching rule is easy to enforce for international staff (two MSF staff were found to be 'intimately touching' and sent home on the next plane out of Freetown) - they are only in the country for a limited period of time. But what do you do for national staff? They have wives and husbands and children. The no-touching rule is limited to non-family members for these long term heroes.

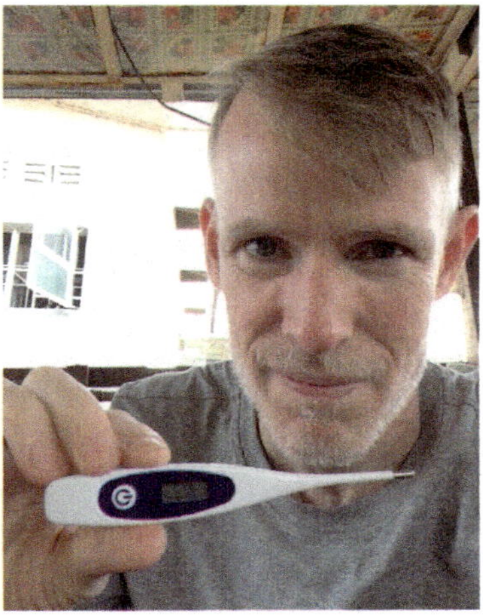

If the staff are suspected of having Ebola then it's straight to admission and isolation (a grim destination). For international staff there is a 48 hour escape rule - if you think you have been exposed then you have a 48 window to travel back to your country before you are at risk of infection. Any possible exposure and you pack your bag, get taken to the airport and catch the next plane out.

But what happens if it's not Ebola? What happens if you have suspected appendicitis? The hospitals have become plague villages, transmission centres for the disease. If you can persuade the staff member to go there, then it's unlikely anyone will go near you. Too many surgeons have died from operating on Ebola patients and their surviving colleagues will not enter the same room as a suspected case let alone wield a scalpel.

I have made friends with the children living next to my guest house in Bo. They are always hanging around as their school closed months ago. Now when they see me returning they rush out full of joy and excitement and hug me, grabbing my hands and dancing with me. What a terrible dilemma - I can't tell them to stay away. I join in the excitement and cover up my discomfort. I ask Joanna, age 6, what she knows about Ebola.

"Never touch anyone sick, wash your hands in chlorine water, if you suspect person has Ebola then call 117, and always do what the Well Body Ministry tells you' she recites in a sing song voice. I like the last bit - always obeying what the Ministry of Health tells you. I'll bring this back as a suggestion for the NHS.

Today we get handed over the keys for our Ebola Centre from the Royal Engineers. 17 truck-loads of medical supplies has left Freetown. We have three days to unload them and to fit out our hospital, but this is for our logisticians. Tomorrow I get my first clinical experience in the red zone.

Saturday, 6 December 2014
First Clinical Experience in an Ebola Centre

At last, my first clinical experience in an Ebola Centre. After the storm of problems setting up our Ebola Centre in Moyamba, the actual clinical job of looking after patients felt like a precious calm. The donning of PPE (personal protective equipment) was less rigorous than the way I had been trained, and all the MSF equipment is different from our UK equipment, but the principles are the same – absolute protection.

My initial nerves over getting dressed up for real for the first time quickly settle as we stride out in pairs into the red zone for our medical ward round. The flow of Ebola Centres is one way – from suspect ward through to confirmed wards and finally the convalescence ward and out. The suspect tent is empty but for two crying children, about 18 months and 4 years old, prisoners in makeshift cots of upturned plastic tables with cheap orange fencing wrapped around the legs to form the walls. Their mother had been admitted to the confirmed ward the day before but they were afebrile, so while the children are likely to have been infected, they were not Ebola cases yet, so could not follow her. Abandoned suddenly and incomprehensibly they were crying helplessly their hearts out for her.

The four year old takes one look at us – scary monsters in our biohazard uniforms – and doubles his efforts, streams of (probable Ebola rich) nasal mucous pouring down his malnourished body. The 18 month old is still too young to be put off by our alien appearance, and holds up both her hands to me, pleading for human contact and love. I hold her hands and she desperately tries to climb up the fencing into my arms. Her crying stops, but only until we walk on, when the duet of misery starts up once more.

The main confirmed wards are surprisingly familiar to me from my African hospital experience. Some patients are sitting outside in the fenced off area, some sitting in their beds, the sicker lying curled and immobile. There is more evidence of diarrhoea and vomiting, the lethal vehicles for Ebola, on the floors and in the buckets. However this was not House-type medical mystery – most of the patients require simple nursing care: pain relief, fluids, antiemetic's.

One corner of the ward houses a family of five, both parents and three children. All but the mother are very dehydrated and severely ill. I put my first IV line in and start to resuscitate the father – for all the cautious training about putting in IV lines as part of my army training, it is surprisingly reflexive. IV lines are not left up between rounds as the patients are confused and inevitably pull them out, so each visit over the Ebola fence provides a chance for a quick life-saving bolus of fluid.

In the convalescent ward a 4 month pregnant mother is awaiting discharge having been confirmed to be clear of Ebola. However, her unborn child is sadly doomed. The concentration of the virus in the placenta spells certain death, and the toxic amniotic fluids of birth are a public health threat to her family. She is facing a bleak choice of a medically induced termination of her baby while still under medical care, or to stay on at the Ebola centre for 5 months until natural birth but with the same inevitable outcome. How do you explain these choices to a young woman who has escaped death herself?

After half an hour in the PPE I feel like I am in an out-of-control sauna. My goggles are fogging up and my vision is impaired. After an hour I have a pounding headache and sweat is literally pouring down all my body and filling my boots which squelch when I walk. My mask is wet with sweat which creates a feeling of drowning. I start putting an IV line in a severely dehydrated five year old, but am thick fingered from double gloves, seeing out of a steamed up window, so do the right thing and pass it over. I last an hour and a half on my first trip over the Ebola fence, much longer than I had expected, my discomfort distracted by the work involved. However, it is still just mid-morning and I dread to think what the rounds are like in the African afternoon heat.

With relief I head to the doffing area knowing that this ritual is going to add another 15 minutes. The doffing monitors are the Kings of the Ebola Centres. They have no qualifications and little literacy, but in the doffing station they have all the power. With chlorine sprayers on their backs like Ghostbusters, these are the guys who will decontaminate me and make sure I am not exposed to any of my heavily exposed protective suit. I am pretty stoical normally but now I am feeling completely shit. The monitor is shouting at me and ordering me what to do: "wash your hands, head back, turn around, wash your hands, outer gloves off without touching outsides, undo your gown strap; gown off; stop! don't touch your hood; wash your hands; gown off; slowly! wash your hands; close your eyes; lean forward; goggles off; dip them three times in chlorine; wash your hands; break your hood ties, all four; lean, wash your hands; remove your hood; wash your hands; undo your gown; stop! don't touch the outside; unzip; wash your hands; remove tape from legs; wash your hands; pull off gown over boots; stop! don't touch your boots; wash your hands; step out of the gown and push to me for spraying; wash your hands; lean forward and close your eyes; remove your mask; wash your hands; step forward for boot spraying." I stagger over the demarcation into the green zone like an exhausted long distance runner, my surgical scrubs drenched with sweat but relieved to have been guided down to land by my very bossy monitor.

I rehydrate and then observe the rest of the ward round in the clinical station, picking up ideas for Moyamba. There is a major challenge in how we communicate the information we collect in the red zone to the green zone. It is difficult to write in PPE, and no documentation can leave the red zone, so MSF have come up with a numeric system for each patient (Patient 001; Bed C3; 1= fever, 2 = bleeding 3= vomiting etc) to shout out clinical updates to a scribe in the green zone. It reminds me of the old jokes of prisoners being so familiar with jokes that they just use numbers. I restrain an urge to make a number up.

Sunday, 7 December 2014
Treatment Trouble in Laka

I feel guilty for not being back in Moyamba where convoys of trucks continue to arrive to fit out our Ebola hospital. However I have settled in to a simple life in Bo. In my house I find an old travel guidebook to Sierra Leone, which informs me that Bo is the country's second city and the nightclub capital - 'Sierra Leone's Manchester to Freetown's London'. Like the Specials song goes, all the clubs have been closed down, and the Chinese-built stadium lies grandly empty. There are no public gatherings now, no parties, no football matches. This is a self-imposed curfew.

Living and working with a local community gives me my first chance to get to know Sierra Leoneans. I have escaped the endless NGO/WHO/Ministry meetings and settled back down to earth. I am greeted with great warmth wherever I walk - sometimes in Arabic, mostly in English. This is a country that loves England more than the English do. Three lion shirts are worn by all the young men, BBC World Service calls out from the transistor radios under corrugated metal roofs, union jacks cover beat up taxis. I am touched with the joie de vivre and resilience of this people. It is a cliché, but happiness bears little relationship with wealth - despite the harshness of people's lives; the daily routines of carrying water and firewood to drink and provide heat, the legacy of the civil war, the new Ebola onslaught. As I stand in the middle of the main street I am immersed in a gallery of smiles and a concert of laughter. While our global market economy would love them to yearn for the latest fashions or the newest smart TV, these are people quietly content with their lives, friendships and loves.

At the Ebola hospital I ask Medlin, one of the clinical officers, about the impact of Ebola on his life. International health workers like myself will come and go, rotating for a few weeks, maybe a few months. However, he has been working on the frontline from the start and will stay until the end. He tells me how he rationalises his risks with the benefits to his community. How he has become a leper to his friends and family who stay away in fear of his direct daily link with the Ebola menace. He lies to his mother about his prestigious job. I ask him if any of his health colleagues have had Ebola and he reels off a football team of names of classmates and co-workers (one just last week) who have died from Ebola as a result of their exposure in health care centres. It is tragic.

Meanwhile, there is trouble at t'Ebola mill. All but one of my 12 NHS colleagues working with the Italian NGO Emergency at Laka have resigned. I wrote about Emergency in an earlier blog - a noble philosophy of offering Western standards of medical care to Africa, but one I felt was mis-guided. Apparently, my colleagues feel so too, and have revolted over the blanket interventional approach given to patients - catheters, IV lines, central lines, toxic drugs injected into all of them, even though many just need a compassionate end-of-life care. Interestingly the mortality rate in Bo (45%) with their very conservative management approach (only 10% get IV lines) is a lot lower than Laka (est. 60-70%).

In Bo they spray your feet with 0.5% chlorine in addition to the 0.05% hand washing routines. As I leave my shift at the Ebola centre I look down and notice that the bottom of my trousers have Jackson Pollock bleached patterns all over them - ah, I remember when I used to do this deliberately. As I am admiring my neo-punk legwear a large rat scurries across the path right in front of me. Behind me Ebola, ahead of me Lassa, it's the devil and the deep blue sea of viral haemorrhagic fevers. My daughter plays an endless game of 'Would you rather…' but this choice is easy - Lassa for me, and so I step forward rather than back.

Monday, 8 December 2014
Ebola Hospitals: High Security Prison for Germs

A late shift yesterday for my final first-hand experience in the red zone before we open Moyamba. The white Ebola ward tents are baked by the mid-afternoon African sun and I manage only 45 minutes in the protective equipment, surfacing for air in the green zone like a diver out of oxygen. There is a danger of a machismo when it comes to the time spent in the red zone. Recently two international health workers were sent home for breaching rules and spending two hours in PPE - a dangerous and unnecessary amount of time.

We see two new admissions transferred by ambulance drive from Moyamba, a three hour drive away. In a week's time we will have beds ready to avoid this long and uncomfortable dislocation. The whole Ebola hospital, with its security fencing and white tents resembles a concentration camp, and the new patient's first contact with us must reinforce that sense of prison visiting. This is a High Security prison for germs with concentric fortifications of chlorine baths and sprays to ensure not a single germ enters or leaves.

From a safe distance we take a picture of the transfer notes that the ambulance driver holds up to his window using a mobile phone, then transcribe them to our own records before a short clinical history. The initial triage involves an interview conducted across two fences, two meters apart. Two nurses then enter in full PPE to guide them through our one-way Ebola maze to the wards. Our hygiene team spring into action with sprayers to decontaminate the back of the ambulance, while the driver sits in his enclosed cabin looking very nervous about his latest fare. There is a well-rehearsed ritual for this decontamination procedure which we will have to practice next week.

We don PPE and follow the patient in. On the ward we carry out a cursory examination and explain the importance of eating and drinking. A standard recipe of antimalarials, antibiotics, analgesia, multivitamins, zinc and anthelminthics are prescribed to everyone. Then it's on to complete urgent tasks, making the most of our dive into the red zone. IV medications for two severely unwell girls. More fluids for patients managing to drink. A check on a young boy who had been convulsing.

I pass by Patricia, the five year old girl I had seen the day before, to see how she is doing. She is dead. Four hygienists in their PPE uniforms spray her body and her death bed, then carefully package and seal her in a white plastic bag, covering everything in a mist of chlorine. Her small, frail body packaged like a postal delivery. Death, a child's death in particular, is an event that you never become desensitised too, whatever your experience, and the excitement of my first front-line experience evaporates in an instant. Her sealed corpse will be exchanged in another complicated decontamination dance to the safe burial team outside the Ebola centre before being dropped in an unmarked grave. All her possessions will be burnt. In a few hours no trace of her short life will remain.

Our break away from Moyamba has provided valuable clinical experience and a rest from the relentless pressure, but time is running out and we must return to prepare the stage for our first patient. Seven weeks of work to do, seven days to do it.

Tuesday, 9 December 2014
A Little Less Action, A Little More Conversation

Our Ebola Treatment Centre is looking perfect for our handover from the Royal Engineers. It's a hospital, built in 7 weeks in the middle of the African jungle. We have a tour around our new home looking for snagging, a couple of short speeches and then its straight to work. Except it's not. One of the challenges of this multinational enterprise is that coordinating several different NGOs and several different national groups is complex. I start to have a deep sympathy for those working in the European Commission.

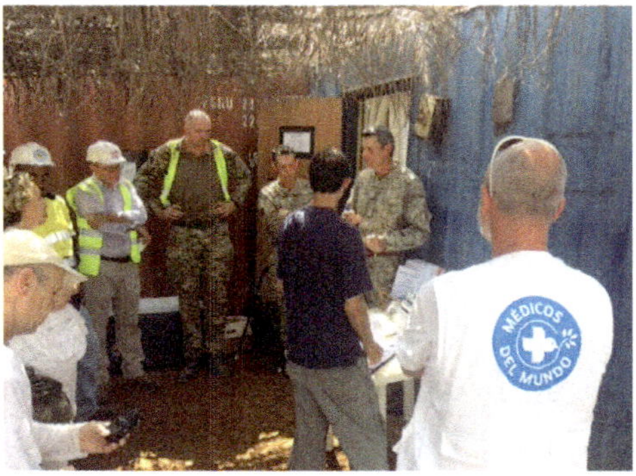

We have our first senior management meeting and discuss our plans. Already, there are suggestions that we postpone the opening by two days until the 17th, perhaps start training in three days' time instead of tomorrow. I control an urge to scream and negotiate a training start date in two days (WHY NOT TOMORROW FOR F### SAKE!!) and a postponement of the opening one day, but I am going to have to heavily sedate my tendency towards impatience. Here we are at the epicentre of the world's worst epidemic and our first senior management action is to announce a public holiday. A little less action, a little more conversation.

The Norwegian team arrive in a flurry of excitement. It is good to be reunited with my Ebola warriors from my army medical training in York. The Norwegian military have delivered their side of the bargain by bringing glamping to Sierra Leone with their very impressive base camp. Five large 8 man tents with air conditioning (!), washing and drying machines (!!), hot showers (!!!), air-conditioned toilet cubicles (!!!!) a kitchen tent with five chefs (!!!!!). This being international aid, not a single penny has been spent in country and everything has been flown in at vast expense from Norway. Even the bottled water, which is a melted iceberg of some sort.

Sadly, the most basic of human needs, internet access, has been overlooked, so we prowl like hyenas around the town, searching for scraps of bandwidth.

One of my key roles is to link the Ebola hospital with the local health services and community, so I decline the St Ebola public holiday and visit the local NGOs we will be working with. Action Control le Faim is a community based NGO with a long track record in the area who will be working with us to support Ebola survivors (if we ever open to have any). All patients have all their possessions burnt as part of the decontamination, so aid packages are offered for a mattress and some clothes. ACF will also be running some of the Ebola ambulances and a network of motorcycle riders who can help with contact tracing and follow up support. Most importantly, they have internet so I luxuriate in the long rambling meeting while my laptop sucks in emails.

Then, to World Vision who will be our partners for those patients who do not survive. They have been running the district safe burial programme for the last few months, and after hearing about the unmarked graves in Bo I am reassured to hear about their approach of respect and compassion. Mr Bundu the burial lead tells me that his team have buried 250 Ebola cases in the last month - every one with a grave marker. This is dangerous and unpopular work, but crucial to the containment of the epidemic. We agree a plan for how we are going to work together to bury our patients who do not survive (if we ever open to have any).

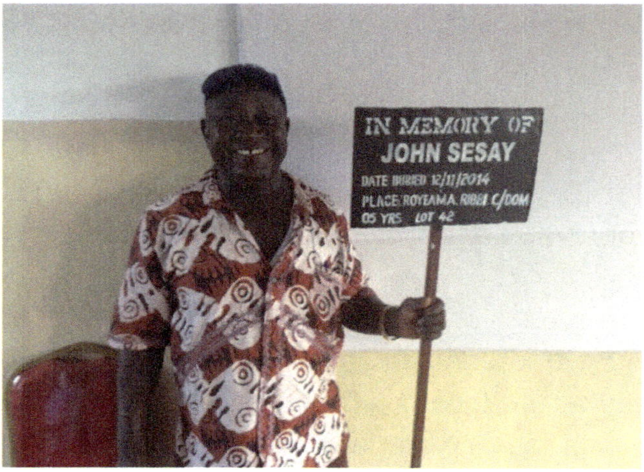
IN MEMORY OF
JOHN SESAY
12/11/2014
LOT 42

Finally, to the Command and Control meeting to hear about the day's latest alerts and confirmed cases. The Sierra Leonean army major in charge welcomes me and I explain how we have been visiting other Ebola hospitals to learn how we can provide the best care for our patients in Moyamba. The audience is enthusiastic until they discover I am also working in the Ebola centre upon which I am informed that the army has strict rules about Ebola segregation, and I will not be allowed to attend future Command and Control meetings. I use science and reason as my allies, but they have UK military advice for their defence, so until I can persuade someone in the command, I am in the farcical situation of being the medical lead for liaison with Command and Control, but barred from their meetings. Maybe I should attend wearing full PPE.

Wednesday, 10 December 2014
Danger of Paralysis by Risk Analysis & Bureaucracy

Induction day and 160 new Sierra Leonean staff and the 12 Norwegians gather in the hanger-like kitchen tent for introductions and then a guided tour of their new home. I take a group of 20 around, sharing their excitement. I ask if any of their families have had Ebola and three of them put their hands up. One woman tells me that her family were the first cases in the country, and with 10 dead, almost wiped out.

Jobs are few and far between in Sierra Leone these days and we have been inundated with applications. The country has an extractive economy - mining - but all the major companies have been scared away. Last week a number of the Chinese mining companies still in operation finally pulled out, panicked by the ever increasing threat from Ebola. The only work left is in the Ebola response itself. So there is a desperation for jobs, but also a real desire to join forces in the fight against this disease that is destroying lives and livelihoods.

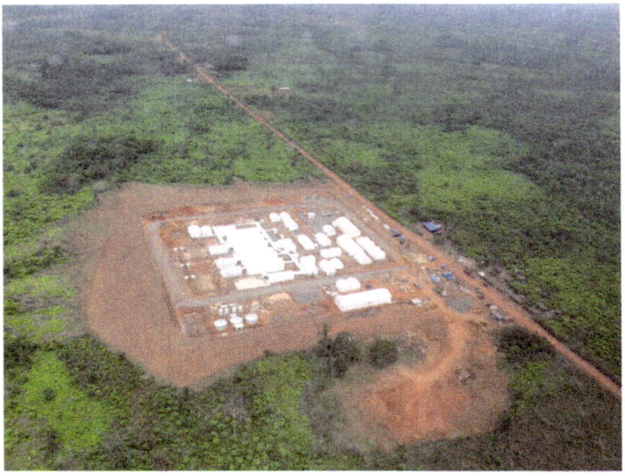

In the hospital the wards are being cleaned and beds lined up. The pharmacy is stocked. There is much training to do and drills to rehearse but our hastily assembled international task force is ambushed with a four-hour long protocol agreement meeting. Item 1a : How to take blood, takes almost 2 hours. Really. So blood from Ebola patients is not something you want to splash around in your face, but we have regressed to the slowest, most cautious pace set by complete risk-avoidance. It doesn't matter that people in the community are dying from Ebola every day, we have to be 100% sure that none of the staff have any chance of exposure. Attaining such absolute safety creates a paralysis by risk analysis and we are in danger of becoming a health and safety orgy. At one stage I start to suspect that this is some sort of cunning plan to bore Ebola to death - “OK humans, I hadn't realised how bureaucratic this was going to be - I give up!”

There is internal wrangling about where the clinical ‘mission control’ office should be, with a suggestion that it is in a small tent far from the red zone. There is a perfect location with great access to triage and the red zone, but if we leave the decision to committee then I am worried we will need a UN convention to agree land ownership, so decide on an old British colonial style. Occupation. While my colleagues drift off into gentle slumber I slip away unnoticed, assemble a few willing volunteers and start moving supplies into the room. By the time the protocol meeting has reached Item 2d: How to pass a sample to the laboratory, we have a respectable clinical briefing room.

The supplies tents that I raid are Aladdin's caves. DfID have sent six sea containers worth of equipment including enough to stock a small NHS hospital, a Boots pharmacy and a Staples store. Two months ago some mandarins in London must have sat down and worked out a list of everything that might possibly be needed and then procured and shipped it. All we really need is some oral rehydration salts and some paracetamol, but the contingency planning is impressive. I climb in large crates and unwrap box after box, like a child on Christmas Day, ending up with that same feeling of emptiness that comes from material overindulgence.

I am worried about the politics of our loose international alliance which really needs a strong, quick-acting dictatorship rather than gentle, slow-witted consensus. One of my Norwegian colleagues tells me that they have a saying in their language: many cooks, much mess. Snappier than our equivalent I feel. I am also a bit worried about the mental health of some of the team - levels of manic anxiety are in the red, and my attempts to reduce them ('just take a chill pill') don't seem to be helping.

At the evening Command meeting I am informed that the national policy, set with UK guidance, is that I will not be allowed to attend the meetings once I enter the red zone. I neglect to tell them that I have already been working in the red zone and protest vigorously: what is the scientific basis for this leper-like exclusion (I am religiously monitoring my temperature); how are they going to integrate practically with our Ebola hospital if they have no representative? What statement are they making by stigmatising health care workers? As a white male I savour my niche discrimination, and am offered an olive branch of a military report to Freetown to reconsider the policy.

Thursday, 11 December 2014
A New Jerusalem in the Heart of a Dark Satanic Plague?

During the last three weeks I had a clear image in my head of the days leading up to the opening of our little hospital in the bush. This was a cross between the efficiency of a BMW factory and the happiness of the seven dwarves. With joyful hearts and steeled muscles we would build this new Jerusalem in the heart of the dark satanic plague.

Inevitably, the reality is a little different. Our barren facility is a post-apocalyptic setting around which we wander dazed and confused under the burning African sun. On the first day we are zombies, staggering from one empty shell of a building to another, overawed by the size of the task ahead of us, clueless about where to begin. We have no water or food and by early afternoon everyone seems to have disappeared, retreat having been decided on as the best form of attack.

By the second day however, we begin to rebuild our civilisation from ground zero. Small groups of nurses cluster together and start to rehearse drills: admissions, drug rounds, rehydration, a collapsed, bleeding patient, a collapsed member of staff. This is a complex adaptive system which is too difficult to design from the top down. It needs to be built in small sections from the bottom up and then assembled in a final grand finale. This empowerment of the staff brings relief and confidence after a couple of days of doubt and concern. I think we can do this.

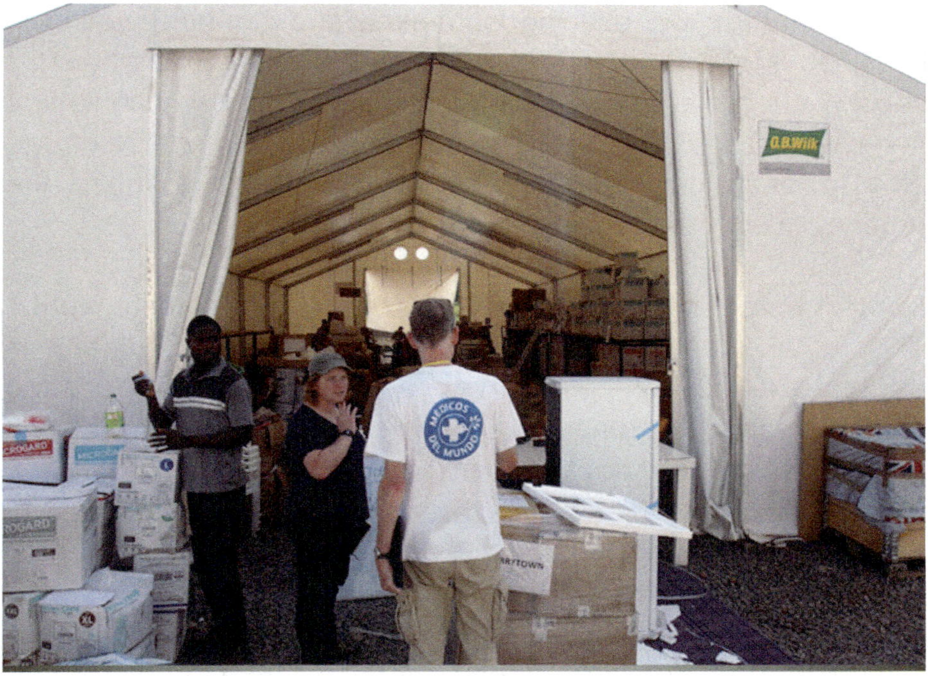

Then again maybe we can't. I get the news from our logistician that we have no gloves, no masks and no surgical scrubs. So maybe I'm a little gung-ho when it comes to pitching into battle with Ebola, but a wafer-thin plastic apron feels a bit naked after all the PPE I have become accustomed to. Trucks of supplies continue to roll up in clouds of red dust from Freetown, but finding what we need is a challenge. Searching for an IV cannula in a lorry-load of crates is literally and figuratively a needle in a haystack.

I call in the offer of help from the Head of the UK Task Force and five minutes later have the promise of next day supplies by helicopter if necessary, and additional army logistical support to help us with the tsunami of supplies. DfID are under a lot of political and media pressure back home, but in country they are guardian angels.

The news from the evening Command and Control meeting is not good. Moyamba town has managed to avoid Ebola by strict security checks at every entrance point. Yesterday it had its first five cases. The Sierra Leonean army has quickly sealed off the area for quarantine, but the Ebola wolf is at the door and the urgency of our mission could not be greater.

Captain Fefegula ends the evening briefing with sombre words. This is like a fight against terrorists and the warfare is asymmetric: every time we are attacked and send reinforcements, the enemy has melted away. We must work harder, and the reward of our hard work will be more hard work.

Friday, 12 December 2014
Conspiracy Theories & Community Engagement

Conspiracy theories swirl around every society, but never more than rural African ones. When I was working in Southern Africa in the 1990s the local young men were adamant that AIDS was a pro-celibacy conspiracy: American Invention to Discourage Sex was their take on the acronym. So it's not surprising that crazy myths and rumours about our Ebola hospital have already started. At the morning Command and Control meeting we are informed that local people have been told that a new hospital has been built to deliberately infect people with Ebola. Apparently a white man has been seen at the Ebola hospital giving people Ebola injections. All thirty people turn to look at me, as I am the only white man in the room, and I can't but help feeling guilty – it's my natural state from a Catholic up-bringing. I try to laugh it off, but end up making a semi-apologetic alibi (IT WASN'T ME, I WASN'T THERE!!)

I decide that some community engagement is needed – to quash the conspiracies but also head off the problems that Kerrytown had being swamped with patients on the first day. I head to Moyamba radio station and offer an interview. Everything is Ebola – the jingles, the songs, the public information announcements. I get my messages across and field a few tricky questions (how many tropical diseases are there in Sierra Leone? What date will Ebola be eradicated?)

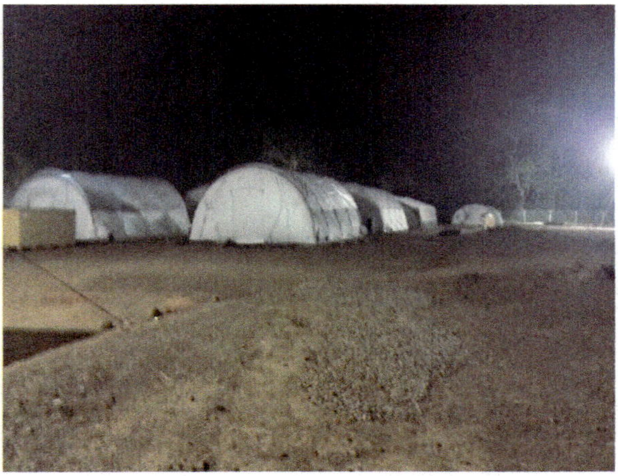

Back at the hospital we continue to fill in the big empty spaces and prepare our routines. It feels too slow for me, but there is much enthusiasm and I enjoy getting stuck in with the local porters as we search through stores and find gems of equipment, as well as less useful boxes. We still have no gloves or masks, though arrival is imminent. I find 500 mobile phones (??) and wonder if rather than donning the PPE we could just give the patients mobile phones and ring them to find out how they are doing in the red zone.

Our evenings are quiet and dull. There is no internet to hypnotise us. No alcohol of course. We eat together on long tables and then the Norwegians have a team meeting, which I am invited to, but as it's all in 'stone-age Norwegian' there is little point. I retire to my tent and write this blog. Then to sleep. I am a light and episodic sleeper. My children are habituated to tip-toeing upstairs after their late nights out to avoid a grumpy dad the next morning. So the communal tent living takes a bit of getting used to. My tent-mates turn-in and rise in different rhythms, with a nocturnal chorus of tossing and turning and snoring and sighs. In the background the most ubiquitous soundtrack in Africa: the chugging hum of the diesel generator.

We are back in our infection control bubble, living in the camp and being ferried to the Ebola Centre three miles away in our own minibus. The Norwegians are forbidden to leave the camp, and I savour my freedom strolling into town. I know you won't have any sympathy with this, but it is very, very hot and even the mildest of exercise exhausts. Oh for some English winter weather.

Things I have learnt today. The Germans pronounce Ebola with the emphasis on the E. The French in contrast pronounce it with the emphasis on the A. In English the emphasis is on the O, though in Yorkshire it will be Eee-bola. Such a short word and so much variation. How strange. The second thing I have learnt today, though unconfirmed, is that one our NHS team has been flown back to the UK with Ebola. Someone I trained with presumably. It is getting closer.

Saturday, 13 December 2014

In town I pass a booming beatbox with a wonderful song about Ebola. It covers health promotion advice about the source (fruit bats and monkeys), the symptoms (shit and vomit, bleeding from your nose), no-touching, what to do when you fall sick, what will happen if you hide sick people (you'll be arrested). And it's a bit of an ear-worm. What a great approach to raising public health awareness

Ola, the team leader for the Norwegians, leaves today. He has been a rock in a stormy time, enthusiastic and wise. We will miss him until he returns in January with the next wave of Norwegian clinicians.

One of the trials of international work is working with other internationals. It can be a cross between Big Brother and I'm a Celebrity, with not- catching-Ebola being this week's jungle challenge. We are a random group of people thrown together in tough and adverse circumstances and expected to get on.

I was interested in observing the British army soldiers interact as they worked and rested 24/7 when there is so little personal space or privacy. They worked hard as a team during the day and in the evening their downtime was quiet and introspected – everyone finding their own emotional space in a packed, cramped basement. These were seasoned professionals doing their job, and with a well-established hierarchy.

In the international camp there are cliques and schisms and blurred hierarchies. Europeans in Africa are stereotypically classified into three groups: missionaries, mercenaries and misfits. We have a few missionaries – not necessarily religious but still hoping to save the world. Since we are all volunteers, I suspect that there are not many mercenaries (though the soldiers could take this mantel). As for misfits – well we definitely have more than our fair share. I'm one of them.

We have splintered into our ethnic groups. Chris and I keep up the stiff British/Irish upper lip, an ethnic minority of two but with a lot of heavily armed countrymen and women living just in case we get persecuted. The Norwegians have safety in numbers, and live up to their taciturn and slightly dull reputation and are good at the camping life. They have sub-divided organically into smaller clusters but age and gender.

The Spanish do their best to annoy the Northern Europeans by dialling up their national stereotype of being loud, late and over-anxious. From the start they decided that shared tents were not for them and have taken over a guest house in town where, rumours have it, there is beer. I am worried that this sends the wrong message out: we are not all in it together, some of us have our own ensuite.

Sunday, 14 December 2014 Moyamba Hospital on the Cusp of Opening

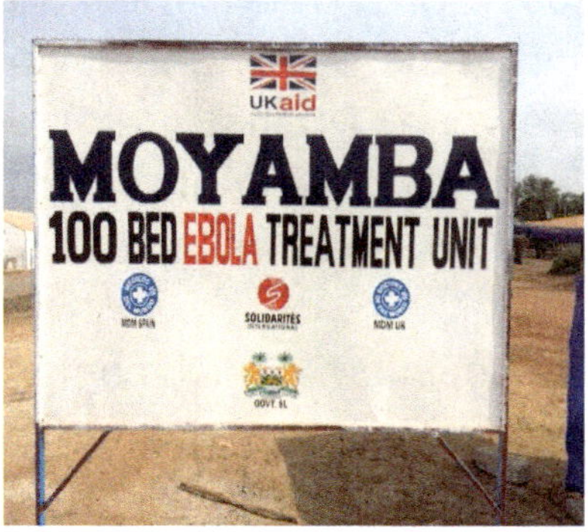

Our Ebola hospital waxes and wanes between storms of activity and lulls of calm. In the intensive phase the wards are full of PPE-clad worker bees swarming around the beds and corridors. Then suddenly, all is quiet as the teams sit in small groups reflecting and adapting the routines. We are still struggling with how to communicate information from our ward rounds. Such a simple task of taking notes on the ward round but unable to take anything out of the red zone. We need information on each patient from our clinical office white board to inform us on the round, and then documentation of any changes from the ward back to the office white board. We consider walkie talkies, but these will corrode with repeated chlorine washes. A microphone under our PPE, but this will get drenched in sweat. Bluetooth or Wi-Fi, but too hi-tech for our low-tech environment and still the problems of chlorine. The flimsy paper checklist used in Bo rapidly becomes damp from all our hand washing and disintegrates. We try small white boards which we carry to the fence and get one of the nurses in the green zone to take photographs, but the distance is too great, even with a zoom lens, to distinguish the words. In the end we laminate sheets of paper which we can soak in chlorine before we take out to the clinical office. It feels clunky, and we need to keep working on this.

Other problems this morning: our body bags leak fluids and so won't be safe to use; our PPE overalls tear too easily and we will need more robust alternatives; the Ebola emergency has now exhausted all the Chinese-manufactured supplies and there is now a global shortage. We will have to beg and borrow from other centres. We have no kitchen equipment yet, so can't cater for staff or patients; our staff toilets have become filthy after just a couple of days and the Norwegians are worried about infection risk; the toilets are flooding because the local contractor used cheap Chinese cisterns; we need to recruit phlebotomists and clinical officers urgently; security is poor at the hospital, particularly at night; we have no chlorine testing kits to test if the concentrations are correct; our goggles are misting up too easily. We have become accustomed to these sorts of challenges and all feel surmountable.

I am trying to improve my community integration with learning a bit of Mende. Before we left the UK we were given lessons in Krio, but Mende is the lingua franca in Moyamba, so I start again. Just a few words of greeting and enquiry brings smiles of amazement to people's faces. A white person who can say "hello"and "how are you?"! Soon everyone is greeting me with a joyful cry of “Dr John!!” and while this is lovely and makes me feel wanted, it also has the downside of having to smile and say hello everywhere I go. No wonder the Queen looks glum most of the time.

Sky News come for a visit. I am pushed forward as the spokesperson. I find that when this happens it is usually because everyone is expecting a disaster and needs someone to be the fall guy. They ask about how we are planning to avoid being another Kerrytown? Have we built too many beds? Why we have built the hospital in Moyamba (subtext: this godforsaken place)? What it's like working on an Ebola ward? There are lots of clinical drills going on which provide good televisual images and we provide a positive picture of the UK's aid effort to combat Ebola, the hospital on the cusp of opening.

Monday, 15 December 2014
Love in a Time of Ebola

Love in a Time of Ebola would be a short sequel. The no-touch rule tends to constrain any amorous tendencies. The whole international aid community seems to have descended on the country and inevitably there are couples working in the same or connected aid projects. The tough decision for these folk is whether to follow the no-touch rules themselves. Some argue that the rule is set to prevent population transmission, so restricting touching to each other creates little risk. Others decide that it is safer to separate so that if one of the couple gets infected, the other will be protected, and they go into self-imposed celibacy and separation.

The no-touch rule is all pervasive, although one of the paradoxes is that teenage pregnancies have shot up. The closure of all the schools has left a generation of school children hanging around their communities, idle and bored. It is not surprising that teenage kicks trump health promotion messages from the Well Body Ministry. The collapse of the country's family planning services, as with all health services, compounds the problem.

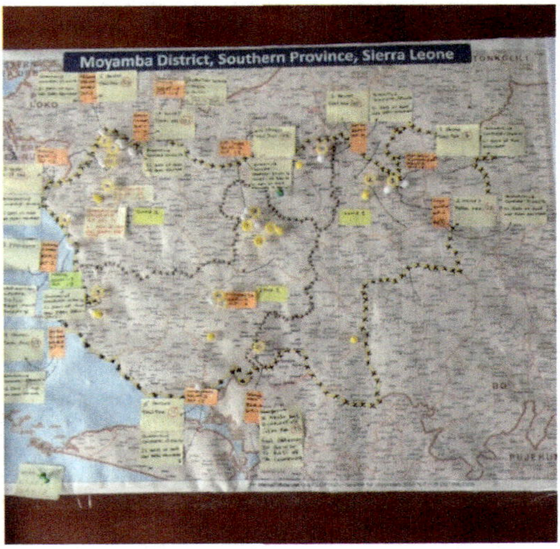

We are making progress at our Ebola hospital, though I fear our opening day is receding slowly. It is now planned for the 17th. Our wards are fully ready for action. Our pharmacy is stocked. Our staff are all trained but now need to have some final dress rehearsals with the infection control teams synchronising with our clinical teams. We are still struggling with our PPE - searches continue around the world for suitable biohazard coveralls. We have even turned to the blackmarket to find what we need. Rather strangely four army Gurkhas turned up at the gate yesterday offering to help and we have put them to work moving equipment and lending shoulders to the final push. A spirit of cooperation has descended on our divided parties and we are all now working to one common goal: our first patient.

Actually a little excitement this morning as we did indeed get our first patient, but sadly/luckily not Ebola related. One of the Norwegian base camp team tripped over one of his sturdily erected tent ropes and dislocated his shoulder. There was a rush of clinicians to help him, deprived of patients for too long and desperate for action. A potent cocktail of midazolam/ketamine/fentanyl and lots of brute force from Chris (who would have thought of an orthopaedic surgeon being the most useful person on our Ebola expedition?) and he has his shoulder back in place, but will be heading home tomorrow.

All the other Ebola Centres have had delays in their openings. If we open on Wednesday we will still be one of the first, having begun the race as the penultimate centres to open. All have had similar challenges of norming and storming between multilateral, multinational partners. There will be many lessons to emerge from this mammoth task about the mistakes we have made. And then at the next global emergency we will repeat them all over again.

Tuesday, 16 December 2014
Ecology of Fear Overtakes Reason: Here and at Home

An early Christmas present from Public Health England. During our training in York we had a very reassuring talk from PHE about how we would not be quarantined on return to the UK. Science would be used to inform guidelines on reintegration with our families and our work. The evidence is clear: if you do not have a fever and are asymptomatic you pose no risk of transmission. So the guidance was that we should take a few days to recover on return at the end of December, then back to work, without risk to patients unless carrying out interventional procedures.

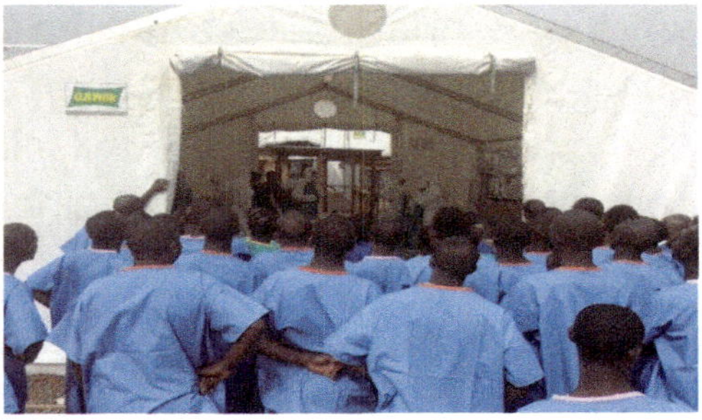

Sadly, the ecology of fear has overtaken reason and the latest guidance has become much more draconian. No travel, no shared accommodation, no clinical work, a fever parole officer to report to daily (yeah, that's going to make the difference), no sex. Hey, where's the bunting and the brass band? Why not issue us with plague masks and bells? I am now trying to work out how I get from Heathrow to home without flying or undertaking journeys longer than one hour. I think if I get off the train at Kings Cross, Peterborough and Doncaster, and catch the next train each time, I will be fully compliant with the guidance. However, I will infect three trains worth of passengers rather than just one (only kidding East Coast Mainline!).

At the Command and Control meeting this evening the army announces that because of the new local outbreak they will start house to house searching in Moyamba to flush out anyone who may be sick. People are hiding their sick partly out of denial and fear of Ebola, but also because they see that they are getting poor care when they are diagnosed. One of our jobs at the hospital is to demonstrate that local patients will get the best possible care available.

Wednesday, 17 December 2014 @ Moyamba District Isolation Centre: The True Heroes of the Ebola War

The opening of our hospital is upon us and it is time to visit the dreaded Moyamba Ebola holding centre where our first patients will be be referred from. In the absence of a treatment centre patients in the district have been quarantined here since the start of the epidemic. The name itself is off-putting with its punitive connotations - containment rather than care being the operative word.

Everyone warns me not to go and I am nervous. Experienced clinicians from other Ebola centres express alarm at the conditions in these 'transmission units' - the fear being that the poor standards of infection control mean they spread disease rather than contain it. However the patients that we will be decanting to our Ebola Hospital when we first open are here, and it's important that we ensure that they are getting good upstream care and not ending up in our triage unit close to death and past medical care. I also want to reassure the nurses working there that we will look after them as we phase the unit out.

When I ask the driver to take me he chuckles and continues driving straight past the junction, assuming that I am kidding. The District Medical Officer offers to meet me outside the unit, but he makes it clear he will not step foot inside. A home-made sign on the wall of what looks like a converted cattle shed announces that this is the Moyamba District Isolation Centre. It has the look and smell of death and neglect. Empty shelves announce the dressing area into the red zone, and no one seems particularly sure about where the low risk area ends and the high risk area begins.

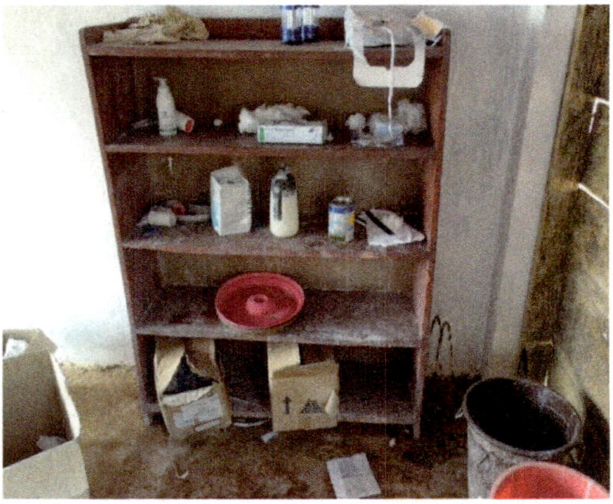

I walk through the main door to find a dark tin-roofed room is furnished by home-made cubicles of plastic sheeting where Ebola patients lie immobile on old rusty beds. It is a room of sickness and fear. There are no drugs, no IV fluids, no medical equipment. The staff have no boots or scrubs, just basic protection equipment. In the backyard blue plastic sheeting and strips of wood have been assembled to create a disinfection area, and a large tent to accommodate those patients who get the all clear. Behind this a brick incinerator bellows the toxic smoke of burning Ebola.

Alfred is the nurse in charge and I enquire about his story. He tells me he was the first person to treat a patient with Ebola at Moyamba Hospital back in April, and he has dedicated himself to caring for these patients ever since. I ask him how many patients he has seen since he set the unit up at the start of August and he methodically counts through his log-book. 220 patients, 120 of them positive for Ebola.

I am stunned and humbled. For five months this decrepit, DIY isolation centre has been on the deadly front line of the battle against Ebola. Every day staff have risked their lives working in inadequate facilities in high risk situations. Then we arrive with great fanfare, 6 months too late, in our fleet of shiny new 4x4s and helicopters, building £2 million worth of Ebola hospital and base camp, staffing it with 200 staff, and prevaricating about the wrong sort of biohazard suits.

I listen to their stories of how they have coped with the infection and death, shunned by their community and the outside world. Amazingly, none of the staff have become infected - testimony to the professionalism of their low-tech approaches to infection control. These are the true heroes of the war on Ebola and I am in awe. I want to swop sides and go and work with them.
I explain how we will gradually start moving patients from the holding centre when we open, and I offer them all jobs at the hospital in recognition of how they have put their lives on the line but also to capitalise on their unique expertise. I walk back to the car conscious that this is the most dangerous place I have been in my Ebola journey. The red zones here and in Bo may be high risk, but with all our protection equipment and infection control facilities they are probably the safest places to be in the current epidemic.

My driver jumps out of the car when he seems me coming. He is edgy and scared. I get a glimmer of insight into the pariah-status that the staff at the holding centre must feel every day. He insists on multiple rounds of hand washing and chlorine spraying of my feet and legs before he lets me back in. We continue our journey in nervous silence.

Back at our Ebola hospital we meet to finalise the opening date. Everyone must agree as safety is paramount. There is one persistent obstacle and that is the PPE. Our risk-averse health and safety lead continues to be paralysed by risk analysis and for 30 minutes we debate small print of different PPE instructions. This is a theological debate where faith triumphs over evidence. Chris and I turn to each other trying to hide our despair. We are going to have to resign ourselves to further delay - now four days from our original start date and getting ever more distant as every day passes.

Thursday, 18 December 2014
It's Opening Day: Almost!

It's Opening Day! I asked the District Medical Officer to come up with a programme and a guest-list, and 24 hours later we have 100 local VIPs including a government minister and press officials. Back home this would take months of preparation because everyone gives the illusion of being so busy with hugely important work, but here in Africa, with casual ease and smooth efficiency we have the perfect, spontaneous celebration.

My attempt to run the event with slick efficiency quickly evaporates as our 10am kick off drifts in-exorably past 11, and our one hour slot for speeches from the local VIPs overflows into three. But this is a big event in Moyamba, so I get into the listening groove and enjoy the long rambling soliloquies. We have a ribbon at the red zone for the local Chief to cut, but he prefers a more traditional ceremony and gets down on his knees to recite incantations and pour water (from a Gordon's gin bottle - it might be gin) on the soil. Then finally, the refreshments and a hubbub of happiness.

Of course it's not really Opening Day. Not quite. One final hurdle persists and that is our biohazard suits (PPE). We now have four types of PPE from DfID. We have hundreds of boxes of the stuff sitting around in our storage tents. However none of them are quite good enough for our quality assurance lead. It reminds me of when I go shopping with my daughters, sitting patiently for hours while they try on all the clothes in the shop, none of them exactly what they are looking for.

Our search is hindered by the global shortage of biohazard suits. The Chinese manufacturers have run out of stock, such is demand in West Africa. Finally, we find a model that passes muster and if our final drills go well today then we are all set to welcome our first guests tomorrow.

Meanwhile, back in the real world of the local Ebola Holding Centre and Moyamba Hospital, our Sierra Leonean comrades are managing to look after Ebola patients whilst wearing flip flops and rubber gloves. The medical superintendent of the local hospital asks me if we have any spare PPE. "How many truck loads do you want?" I reply with festive generosity.

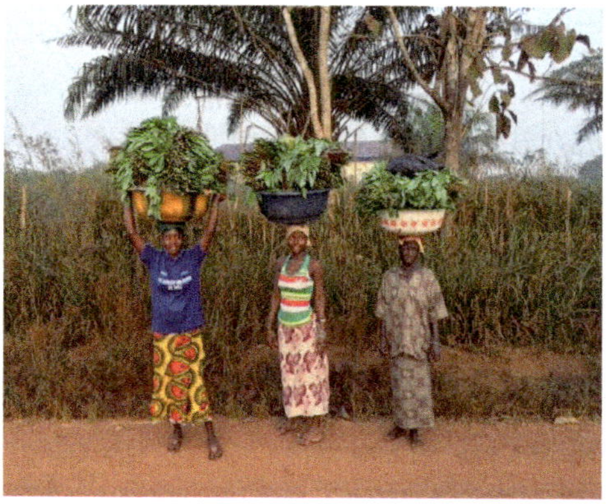

There are concerns that we should not be donating biohazard suits that do not meet our exacting standards, but this is more about legal culpability rather than genuine concern about risk of exposure to local staff. I suggest a convoluted (and spurious) donation system whereby MDM return the boxes of PPE to DfID and I then seek permission from DfID to donate to the local hospital. With no objections I set off in a loaded pickup truck and at Moyamba Hospital I am greeted as an Ebola Santa Claus. Health staff unload the unlikely Christmas presents with excitement and joy. I feel like I have just relieved the Alamo.

At the evening Command and Control meeting I provide a heartfelt apology for the repeated delays and continuing uncertainty about our opening date. One more day! The community expects.

Friday, 19 December 2014
First Patients Safely Admitted

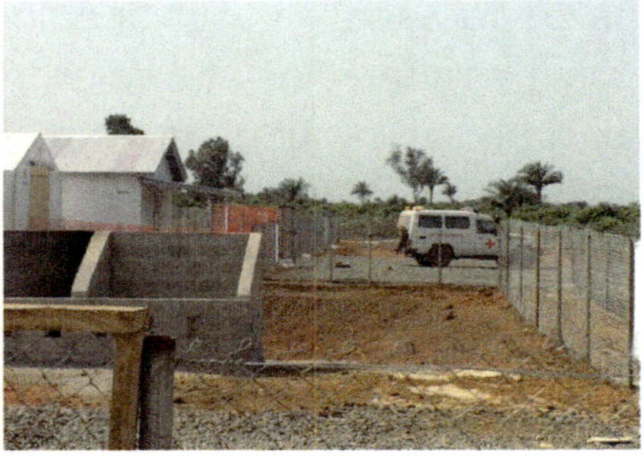

With the planned opening hit by sniper fire on the first day, the rest of the week crawls along on its hands and knees in search of cover. Finally, by Friday the civil war is over and everything is set for our first patient - just four days late, though it feels like four weeks. However, perfection continues to be the enemy of the good, and our infection control team (watsan/WASH/IPC - lots of different names for essentially showering us with chlorine in the red zone) still has final changes and rehearsals that they want to finish before kick off. They agree to stick with the day but want to postpone until 2pm. I offer 10am. They offer 1pm. I offer 11am.

They revert to 2pm. Do they not know how bargaining works? We settle on a 'review at 10am and if all is ready we will admit the first patient at 12 midday approach' although I can tell from the way they avoid my gaze that they are already thinking of another week-long rehearsal.

Off to Command and Control to see if I can engineer a mid-morning referral and then use emotional blackmail to settle the deal. Having worked in the NHS for 20 years I know how to manipulate waiting lists and admissions. Three Ebola-positive patients are waiting for us in the Holding Centre. All are reported to be clinically stable. The group is impatient about the suggested 2pm transfer and I do everything in my power to stir things up as much as I can. Pretty soon the Sierra Leonean army is brandishing AK47s and shouting 'Death to the Medics'. I think I might have pushed things a little too far.

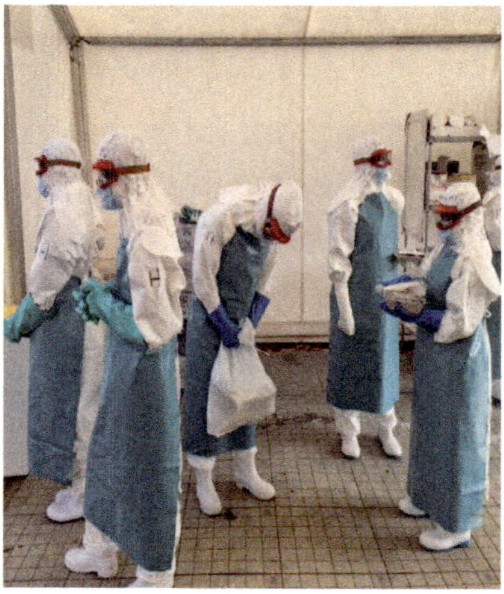

Three stable, confirmed patients are the perfect test for our opening so I rush back the hospital to try to get an early admission, but the best I can do is 1.30. So the patients languish for a few more hours in poor conditions while we rearrange the plastic chairs in the doffing area.

The entire Norwegian team awaits with nervous excitement. This is the moment they have been practicing for six weeks. It's E-Day. Inevitably for our first night performance everything goes wrong. The ambulance drives to the wrong entrance. A group of local health staff drive along behind taking photos of the great occasion, rather morbid tourists, who we have to chase away. The ambulance stands for too long in the mid-afternoon heat while the team dresses in PPE. There is no security guard to open the external gate to get access. But all in all our rehearsals pay off and we have our first patients safety admitted and under treatment.

The three patients are not as stable as we anticipated. All are 4/5 days into symptoms at the critical phase when they can deteriorate rapidly, but they are in the safest possible place. The Norwegian team are desperate for front line red zone action, having waited so long. They get their adrenaline fix and do a great job. There are lots of things we need to improve, but this is really a continuous quality and safety improvement cycle and we will get better and better. We practice the use of mobile phones to take images of the medical notes that cannot leave the red zone and this works well. The patients get their meds and their fluids, a wash and a rest. We have lift off!

Meanwhile, back at our Norwegian base camp we have the Internet. Just a trickle, but enough for emails, and if you are very patient, an occasional glimpse of the web. In the evening we no longer sit around under the African stars sharing tales and cultures. Such carefreeness is replaced with solitary staring into the screens of phones and tablets. Ahhh, it's just like being at home.

Saturday, 20 December 2014
Cookbook Medicine at its Most Simple

Moyamba is Mende for 'Send for Us' and it feels quite appropriate today. The community has asked for help and we have come. We have built and opened this specialist hospital in the middle of the jungle, and now finally, we have patients to care for. The focus on clinical work is a much needed distraction from the sectarian debates about protocols and risk. All the tensions that have been running between the different camps melt away and there is a mood of achievement and celebration.

Chris and I have taken to walking across town each morning, along the dusty red roads to the Ebola hospital. This army of 30 Europeans descending on the town must seem threatening, and our transport, like American presidential convoys, appear elitist. So walking gives us a much needed opportunity to engage - to talk and laugh and share with local people, to play with the curious children. The town clings to a long-forgotten colonial past when the railway ran through the town on the way to mines to the East. Crumbling grandeur is mingled with mud and wattle homes. Goats graze on the verges and dogs chase chickens across the road (the answer to the perennial riddle).

Pride of place in the central cross-roads lies a crumbling tower of concrete, worn away by the elements so it has become almost Gaudi in its form. At each of the corners an orange lion stands guard with a gurning, smirking face. The sculptors most have had great fun building this civic monument.

I am worried about a quasi-apartheid in the hospital. Our senior management team is all white, and our clinical office has become the preserve of the Norwegian clinicians. It is so critical that we tap the wisdom and expertise of the national staff and move rapidly to putting them in charge. However, the structure of our international invasion excludes any Sierra Leonean co-production, and there is a vested interest to maintain the status quo. My efforts to make steps towards real integration are met with unanimous agreement, but nothing happens.

I do the dawn ward round on our three patients who lie on their 'Britishaid' hospital beds, dwarfed and lonely in our neat row of circus tents. There is a pattern of symptoms from Ebola that is quickly recognisable. Our patients have extreme exhaustion, dyspepsia, nausea and diarrhoea that is typical. The older woman, Saffie, is conscious, but barely able to sit up. IV fluids and antibiotics are having little noticeable benefit. Her age is against her in this life and death race. The younger patients are stable, but need better pain relief and more fluids. This is cookbook medicine at its most simple. With our biohazard suits and fear of contagion it is easy to forget to be human and I make an effort to hold and embrace them, to show some compassion, to share their suffering.

There are still teething problems. Using goggles are a nightmare - after 5 minutes in the red zone our vision is seriously impaired, and clinical procedures become games of blind man's bluff. There must be some international consensus to move to face visors quickly. MSF apparently won't change from goggles to visors mid-epidemic and WHO, who are supportive, have less credibility due to their late entry into the epidemic. In the meantime we stagger through the high risk red zone in a Sottish mist, our heads held back to catch a glimmer of vision at the bottom of the lenses where the water pools. We try anti-fogging agents, toothpaste, spittle - but to no avail. Our double-glazed masks seem to hinder any solution.
Our kitchen is still not operational, but our cooks just revert back to traditional cooking techniques and are soon rustling up spicy fried rice for the patients breakfast and the staff lunch.

Back in town everyone is busy cleaning their yards and sweeping their houses. The President has announced a national cleaning day as part of the 'defeat Ebola' efforts. I express surprise about the degree of compliance, but am told that those who disobey face arrest.

One of my MSF colleagues explains about the unprecedented global response to Ebola. “You don’t bring home famine on the sole of your boot”

Sunday, 21 December 2014
Ebola: A Terrible Disease, an Unpredictable Grim Reaper

Ebola is a terrible disease. The pain, fever, exhaustion, confusion, diarrhoea and vomiting creates a carpet bombing attack on the human body. Our three patients dip in and out of this grim journey, and the unpredictable course of their illness is unsettling. They are all still alive, but demonstrating the rapidly fluctuating symptoms typical of Ebola.

Saffie, the older women with a poor prognosis has, against expectations, improved considerably from her near-moribund state yesterday. Isatu, the younger woman, deteriorated yesterday and we ramped up treatment with some signs of hope. She is well enough to talk and we find out that she is less afraid of dying from Ebola than the consequences of what this will mean for her children. She is separated from her husband and has ten children. Her five month old daughter died last month but the other children are now abandoned at home with no one to support them. She cares little about her suffering and pain, distracted by her concern for her children. Ladybird, ladybird.

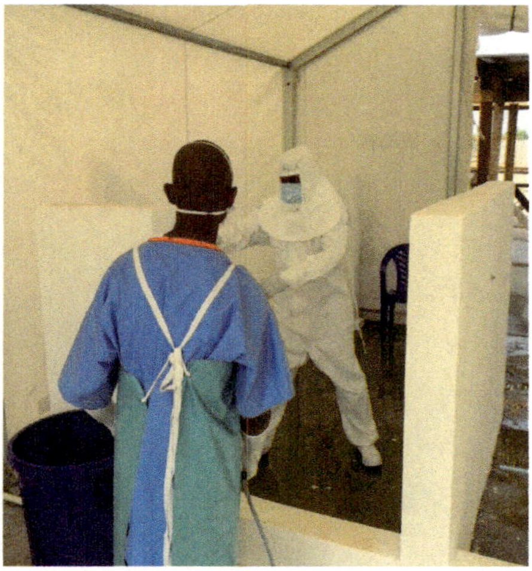

Ibrahim, the younger man, was eating and drinking yesterday and the one we were least worried about. However, overnight he has deteriorated rapidly and is now demonstrating neurological symptoms, a bad prognostic sign. He is confused and almost catatonic, the zombie-like state of late Ebola, and seems to have some symptoms and signs of meningism. It is important that we do not exclude other co-morbidities, though we have little we can do to investigate other causes - our one and only lab test is Ebola PCR. The three patients have been jostling for position in the critical list, but today it is Ibrahim who is most likely to die.

On the afternoon ward round I find him unresponsive. It is difficult to feel a pulse with the double gloving and difficult to check his pupils with my fogged up goggles, but it doesn't take long to conclude that he is dead. Our first Ebola fatality. I stretch out his arms and legs, and cover him with a blanket. Early signs of rigor mortis are already beginning. He may have been dead for an hour, maybe two, but we are dependent on our smash and grab dashes into the red zone, so it is impossible to be certain of the time of death. The chlorine sprayer is twitchy as she washes my hands and she drops her sprayer. She knows that Ebola is most dangerous at death, and she is scared of the body, and after my close contact, she is fearful of me.

A sudden sadness descends on the team after a day of joy from the opening. Ibrahim was young and fit and almost symptomless on admission, the clear favourite for survival. One day later he is dead. Ebola is an unpredictable grim reaper.

The rest of the afternoon is spent trying to find out how to get hold of a death certificate, and trying to liaise with the safe burial team. We have to contact the family, but they live many miles away and we have no such thing as social services. I quickly appreciate how disconnected our upstart facility is from the community and the established social systems.

The plan for all the Ebola centres is to open with a small number of patients and test the resilience of the facility and the staff routines. 36 hours after admission we are confident about how we are managing and it is time to scale up. Meanwhile I have my first resident night on call in over 20 years.

Sunday, 21 December 2014
Festive Boot Christmas Trees

Christmas is coming. It is a time of families and friends, of giving and sharing, of joyfulness and celebration. Here we are in Moyamba, isolated in the middle of the African jungle, thousands of miles from home, separated from our loved ones, and, inevitably, we all have one thing on our minds: alcohol.
The prohibition of the Norwegian camp may be great for our minds and our bodies. But it does get a bit dull, and a sign of how desperate things are getting is that we are struggling to recall what beer tastes like. The only alcohol we have had for the last month has been the hand gel that we use in our repetitive daily rituals.

The British army forward operating base (FOB) is still at the disused stadium in town and the hospitable young captain kindly invites Chris and myself round for a traditional Christmas dinner. They will be on 24 hour stand down and for the first time in months allowed (at the captain's discretion) to buy alcohol. The Brigadier is threatening to do a helicopter visit of all the FOBs on Christmas day, but this will involve half the crew of HMS Argos remaining on standby in case something bad happens and so there is mutiny in the air. Plans are afoot to change the name by deed poll from Argos to Bounty.

I mention our army invitation to the Norwegian camp commander who immediately rises to the national challenge and offers to have a 24 hour stand down at our camp with more alcohol than the army. I don't know how much alcohol the army will have (there are only six of them left now), but I have no doubt that in this escalating alcohol race of mutually assured drunkenness, the Norwegians will win.

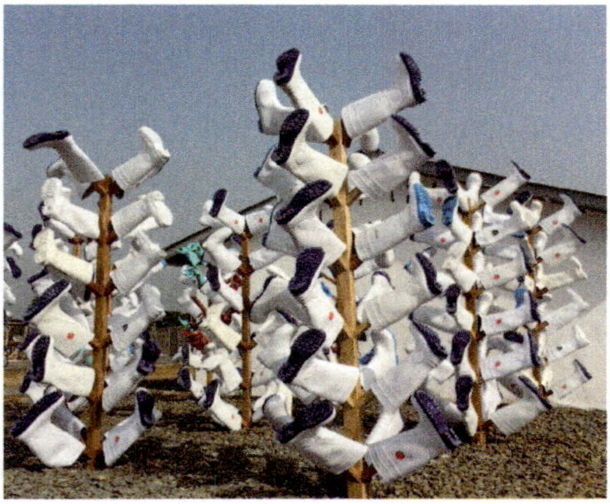

Fortunately a solution emerges. The Norwegians celebrate on Christmas Eve (Yule) and the British on Christmas Day. Brilliant. Run the two 24 hour stand downs sequentially and we have 48 hours of drinking. Although work might just get in the way a bit. I will be resident on-call on Christmas Eve so may end up missing both our first alcohol day through abstinence, and the second through fatigue.

ACF, one of the local NGOs is thinking of having a Christmas party. This suggestion generates much excitement in the camp, but not due to the anticipation of great company and food. ACF have been in Moyamba for a number of years and, importantly, have a satellite dish and very good internet. I suspect they will not be overly impressed when we all turn up with our laptops at the ready and sit around in silence catching up on Facebook.
s
Meanwhile the Norwegians have pushed their Viking boat out with the Christmas decoration(s) and we have decided that our surgical boot drying trees look particularly seasonal for festive celebrations!

Monday, 22 December 2014
Patience for patients

At night the Ebola hospital looks like the circus has come to Moyamba. There is little electricity in the town and our illuminated tents and security lighting provide a festival of light.

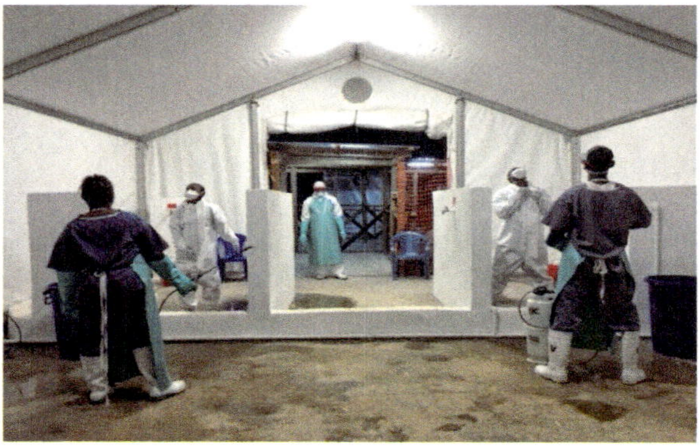

The night shift has a skeleton staff, but with only two patients the staff to patient ratio would be the envy of the NHS. Few patients are admitted during the night in rural Africa - road traffic accidents and obstetric emergencies mostly. On my first night on call I get just one suspect case referred. Unfortunately, the case is a 17 year old who is pregnant. Pregnancy and childbirth is at the highest risk for transmission due to the potential for exposure to viral-rich blood and amniotic fluid during labour. The maxim goes: don't undertake any procedure where you can't see your fingers, which essentially means midwifery becomes a spectator event. The only intervention is sublingual Misoprostol after delivery to minimise postpartum bleeding. Even cutting the cord is viewed as a risky procedure. The baby always dies and the mother usually follows.

It is over 20 years since my last obstetric experience, so this does not seem like the ideal time for a quick refresher. Fortunately, the ambulance makes a mistake and takes her to the government hospital rather than to us. I breath a deep sigh of relief.

We are ghost-like apparitions in our white biohazard suits under the fluorescent lights of the walkways. Saffie has deteriorated after her brief resurgence this morning and I think she is going to die overnight. I am dejected. We have arrived with fanfare and hope and we are failing. We are doing everything we can, but we are losing. We have only two patients, but they are an early test from the community about the difference we will make.

During the night I try to catch glimpses of Saffie from the green zone and return with hope when I see her lift an arm or move her head.

We have 100 beds in the hospital (more realistically 60-70 to avoid the beds being too close to each other in the tents) and earlier in the day we have been discussing how quickly to scale up. The medics are keen to expand rapidly (quelle surprise) but the water/sanitation (watsan) lead is as usual far more cautious and wants to increase capacity by 3 beds per week. We point out that the epidemic will be over by the time we reach full capacity, but we know from the last week that this is not an argument that we will win (we never win any arguments with them). Chris manages to negotiate a peace pact whereby the clinical teams can go in solo without a murmuration of chlorine sprayers swooping around us all the time. This is a real breakthrough.

I am surprised there have not been more suspected or confirmed cases referred to the hospital during the day. The numbers recorded at the Command and Control meetings do seem to be falling in recent days and my next anxiety (my anxieties pass like batons in a relay race) is that we won't have enough patients to fill our empty new beds.

I speculate four hypotheses for the unexpected low numbers in recent days:

1) The epidemic is over. This is my favourite, but probably a little optimistic. While it is my favourite it also sparks a flicker of disappointment. Having put so much into setting the centre up, it feels a bit of a shame not to be able to use it fully. This feeling troubles me as I think I might be Dr Evil.
2) The rapid increase in UK funded Ebola Centre beds in the last couple of weeks is dwarfing demand. The number of beds has doubled from 500 to 1000, and it may be a basic market forces issue: excess supply and diminishing demand.
3) People are hiding their sick relatives. We know this is happening in a number of chiefdoms, especially with Christmas coming. Ribbi in particular, where I will go tomorrow to investigate further.

4) Ebola is taking a bit of a break for Christmas. Perhaps going home to er, Ebola, for the holidays.

Hypothesis 1) is not as far-fetched as it might appear. I hear that the Ebola Centres in Bo and Kenema have been contacting the Ebola response teams to ask for patients, as they have seen patient numbers fall in the last week. Kailahun, the first centre that experienced the Ebola epidemic in Sierra Leone, has apparently discharged its last patient. So it may be that the tide is finally rapidly turning.

Hypothesis 2) has validity as the rapid increase in capacity will be spreading demand. I envisage the new Ebola centres fighting for business in this new competitive environment. I join the fray and start emailing all my contacts in Freetown and national centres to advertise that we are open for business. Maybe some TV advertising.

Hypothesis 3) is also a real concern. House to house searching has begun in Freetown, and tomorrow is begins in Moyamba. The local Chief has decreed (see letter) that the search will be for the sick, the dead, and strangers who are not allowed to stay at home. The sick and the dead will be reported (I'm not sure this threat will work for the dead). We should expect to uncover more cases.

The next few days will be test these hypotheses. On the dawn ward round Saffie is alive and stronger. I dare to hope. Meanwhile, rather sleepily, I am off to confront the rebels of Ribbi.

Our efforts to look after them are hindered by language barriers - none of them speak Mende and our nurses speak little Timini or Shabu, the languages from their home district of Ribbi (see the cool interactive map!)

Tuesday, 23 December 2014
A Trickle of Patients & Safe Burials

The District Medical Team have postponed the trip to Ribbi so I spend the day in Moyamba. With our doors fully open for business we start getting a steady number of suspect case referrals to the Centre. The first is a young teacher who seems to have Ebola but is in the early stages and not too ill. The second is a confused older woman who it is difficult to get any history from and the diagnosis is less likely. She has a nasty wound on her foot and we test her glucose to check for diabetes. She is extremely hyperglycaemic, but we have no insulin to treat her.

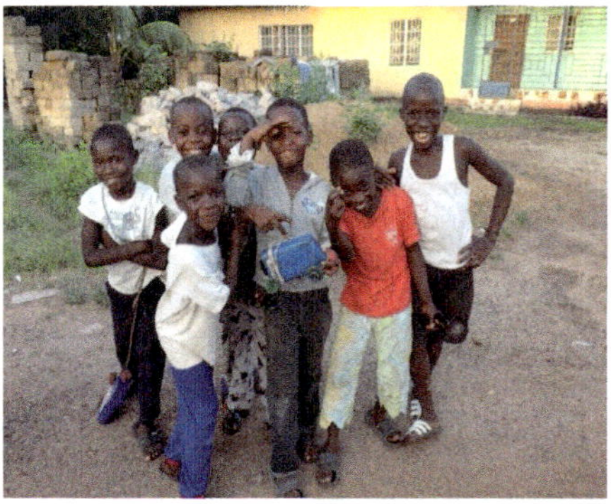

I have asked the Command and Control to be our air traffic controllers and keep us notified of any ambulances but, inevitably, this does not happen and the day quickly becomes chaotic. We are taken completely by surprise when two ambulances turn up in quick succession. It is the second that causes the greatest problem.

I am told that there is a woman in the ambulance. I have no further details, no name, no symptoms, no reason for referral, no notes, just a Landcruiser ambulance parked ominously outside waiting in the mid-afternoon heat with its red lights flashing. We have only just finished with the preceding case, so we quickly start preparing once again. The news then arrives that it is not a woman, but a child with a nurse in PPE in the back of the ambulance. The child is about 10 years old the security guard informs me. Her mother has Ebola.

Our watsan team head to the ambulance docking station and, after careful decontamination, carry the child into the suspect ward on a stretcher. Meanwhile, I dress in PPE with two of the nurses to follow on with clinical assessment. When I enter the four watsans are standing waiting patiently, one at each corner of a stretcher lying on the floor next to a bed. On the adult stretcher lies a tiny two year old girl, silent with fear. There are now seven of us in full PPE in this aircraft hangar of a tent. It is so overpowering, so unequal.

I pick her up in my arms. I know that there is a risk she may pull my goggles, but she is so small and afraid that I cannot resist. She clings to me with the reflex of a toddler, and the stoicism of an African child. She is beautiful.

I ask the accompanying nurse about the child. She knows little. We have no name, no parent, no record, no history. The nurse had been at the primary health care clinic when the child was brought in as an orphan. The story was that her mother had Ebola, and that her mother was here in our hospital. The child has some symptoms, but only what the nurse has witnessed in the last hour.

I can't believe how messed up all this is. We know nothing about this child. She is abandoned in the red zone of an Ebola centre.

Her mother may be one of the patients in the confirmed ward next door, but we can't take her in because we don't know if she has Ebola, and if we do then she certainly will. The story is so unreliable that she probably shouldn't even be here, but there appears to be no where else for her to go, and no one else who will take her with her deadly infection connection. She is a pariah, an Ebola outcast.

We give her some paracetamol and vitamins crushed in some honey. Then some milk. She is not particularly unwell, but will need full time feeding and caring, and our red zone dashes do not allow for this. We have two suspect cases now in the suspect ward, but only one who is alert. I ask the teacher if he could help us - to come to the fence to tell us if she needs our help. We move her cot to the walkway end of the tent so we can see her from the green zone.

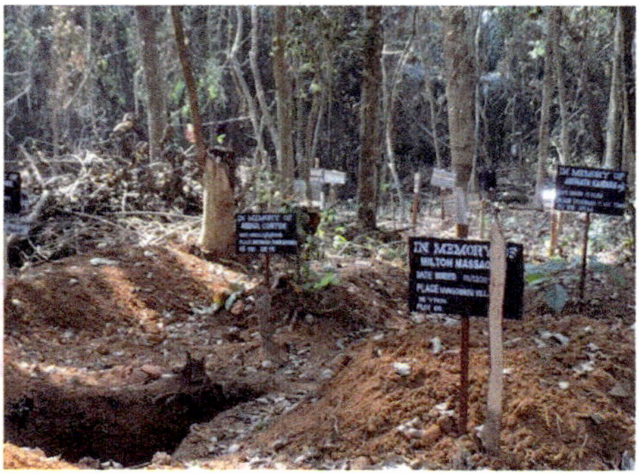

I am tired from my night on call but still have to sort the safe burial for Ibrahim. The law of the country is that everyone must be buried safely (sprayed with chlorine and put in a body bag) within 24 hours of death. Each evening I listen to the list of safe burials in Moyamba, mostly old people and children under 5. These will be deaths unrelated to Ebola, but in this national emergency there is a blitzkrieg approach.

Mr Bundu is the head of the safe burial team and he takes me to the Ebola cemetery. It is a beautiful place, cut out of the jungle on the edge of town. Sunlight dances through the canopy illuminating the neat rows of grave markers. A team of 11 grave diggers prepare more graves, including Ibrahim's. They dig 8 feet down rather than the usual 6 feet. Deep silos for these toxic Ebola corpses.

I hope that it will remain as a memorial when all this is over. Not just for those who have lost their lives, buried where they died, but as a reminder to be vigilant in future, to avoid the tragic mistakes that we made this time in not preventing the epidemic. Lest we forget.

A Presidential Cow for Christmas

The President has given each district Ebola team a cow for Christmas. We are touched. Our cow grazes contentedly outside the Ebola Response Centre HQ. It would make a lovely pet with its large brown eyes, but I fear that by tomorrow morning it will be Christmas dinner.

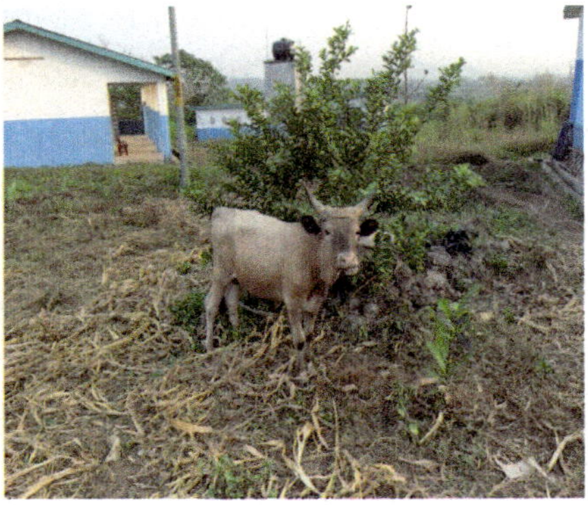

The latest Ebola situation report (I can't get myself to call it the sitrep) for the country is looking very good. Kenema and Kailahun have no patients left. Bo is down to 10. When I was there 10 days ago they had over 50. Chris returns from a meeting in Freetown for all the new DFID funded Ebola Centres and it appears that numbers of patients are low:10-20 per centre. Hotspots remain - in Port Loko and Freetown - but there has been no surge in reported cases following the house to house searching.

My continuing sense is that we are nearing the end of the epidemic. There is genuine societal behavioural change on hand washing and hygiene; nearly all burials are now safe burials; we have plenty of isolation facility capacity now. This war may not be over by Christmas, but it won't be too long afterwards.

A hugely frustrating day yesterday. Our bore holes have run dry, so we have no water. I am sceptical about all our fussiness over different brands of PPE and suspect we don't need most of the well-stocked pharmacy we have, but there is one thing we certainly do need for infection control, and that is water, and lots of it. Recriminations inevitably begin. The local sub-contractor has apparently used cheap and shoddy materials that are already breaking up and the water may just be leaking away. The bore holes dug by the Royal Engineers were fine when they tested them in the rainy season, but now it is the dry season, the water level has fallen, and cannot meet our 24 hour needs. All we need is to find a replacement water supply, but our efforts at finding available water tankers to bring in water are falling on symbolically appropriate dry ground. It is Christmas Eve - this is not a good time to set up a 20,000 litre daily water delivery. I wonder if we can use all the bottled Norwegian water from the camp. Finally, Sandra, our wonderful new hospital coordinator comes to the rescue and we are promised water for Christmas.

Our patients don't know this of course, and ambulances continue to turn up unannounced at the gate, despite my efforts to get prior notification. Without water we have no choice but to turn them away, and back to the heroes at the Moyamba holding centre who manage with a couple of nurses and a cleaner what we can't do with 200 staff. I still hold out hope that they will put in a January transfer window request for me.

It is a good time to take a rare trip out of town, to visit Ribbi district. Of particular interest to me is a visit to the main district town of Bradford, the namesake of the great city where I work as an NHS consultant.

Bradford, Sierra Leone, has been a very naughty town. At the Command and Control meetings there are regular alerts of secret burials and hiding of sick patients. There are reports of illegal gatherings and strangers being allowed to move through the area without being checked. Perhaps not surprisingly the district is also a hotspot for Ebola. Our first three patients were all from Ribbi.

So a surprise raid is planned for Christmas Eve to reclaim the lawless jungle paths of Bradford.

Wednesday, 24 December 2014
A Bumpy Ride to Bradford, Moyamba

The morning Command and Control meeting is packed with increasingly outrageous stories about what the people of Bradford and Ribbi are up to. It sounds like some sort of Dionysian orgy.

Our recon mission to bring order to the lawless streets of Bradford will involve the SL army, police, British army and the district health team. By the time we finish the meeting and break

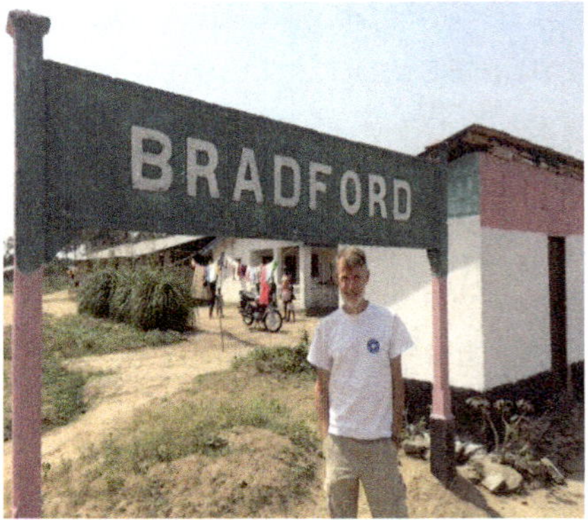

up to head to our convoy of 4x4s we are pumped up into a frenzy of righteousness. Let's do it! Yeah! Booyah! Let's go! The British army contingent have by far the best looking vehicle, so the DMO and myself place strategic reservations for the back seats of their Land Cruiser.

Of course we don't just go. Our 9am departure meanders past 9.30 and then 10. By 11am there is no sign of any imminent departure in fact everyone seems to have disappeared on spurious errands. Eventually, with Western impatience,, the British army team decide to head off, persuading the health team to join us. The SL army and police promise to follow 'five minutes' later.

The road to Bradford is an old British-built railway line, pulled up many years ago, and it is terrible. It looks like something that the Top Gear team would choose for a monster truck expedition. We bump and thud across rocky outcrops and through precariously deep rivers. One day somebody is going to buy this Landcruiser from Autocar and be very disappointed in how the one careful owner has treated it.

We pass through numerous fever and hand-washing checkpoints on the way. I ask one security guard if he gets many cars going past. We are the first he says. I'm not clear if this is just for this day, or forever. The villages are well-kept, many with home-made hands-free chlorine dispensers outside each hut. The social mobilisation team have left their mark and entire communities are living a life of Godly cleanliness.

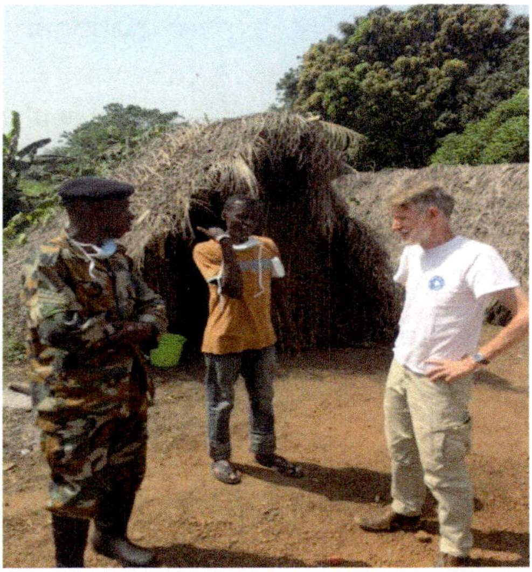

We arrive in Bradford with aching backs and relieved sighs, to be greeted by a well-maintained train station sign announcing our destination. A perfect photo opportunity! Our police and army colleagues end up leaving nearly an hour after us, but roar up in a great cloud of dust within minutes of our arrival. They must have been flying over the ditches and rocks.

Our entourage must be the most exciting thing that has happened in Bradford for months, but the local people are nonchalant and wary of us. I smell disobedience in the dry heat of the midday air. We try to track down the Paramount Chief and are directed to a nearby village. a couple of miles away. Everywhere appears to be ‘a couple of miles’ away in distance, a description that bears little resemblance to reality.

We head off down increasingly remote jungle tracks. Our Sierra Leonean army escort look a fearsome lot, standing menacingly in the back of the military pick up as it bumps up and down. One of them wears an SAS style balaclava in luminescent green. They look like a cross between an ISIS scouting party and a fancy dress party. As we go deeper into bush the thought does cross our minds that this might be well be some elaborate ISIS ruse to kidnap us. It is for occasions like this that as an Englishman I proudly carry my Irish passport.

We end up at a river boundary separating two villages. The Paramount Chief is nowhere to be found, but the two village chiefs are rounded up and with them a crowd of curious on-lookers. The local language is Shabu, so we translate from Krio to Shabu, and when I talk, from English to Krio to Shabu. I suspect Chinese whispers may be altering the content of my speech as they look completely perplexed when I finish. However, the key messages are driven firmly home by the head of the health team. The President is angry; Ebola is a killer; they must change their wicked ways; this British doctor will leave us and go home if they don't (I'm not sure if this a threat or an incentive). Safe burials, good hygiene and no more strangers..

For all the bad reputation that they have built up, they seem unexpectedly compliant and agreeable. The chiefs promise they will behave and we head off along bad roads to continue our search for the Paramount Chief. The army and police escorts appear to think this is a dress rehearsal for a Jason Bourne film, and we struggle to keep up. No wonder they caught us up so quickly this morning. Perhaps not surprisingly after 5 minutes the army pick-up has a puncture. We discover that we have one spare tyre between the three vehicles - the one on our British army Land Cruiser. It takes another half hour while we work out how to release the spare tyre. A large group of men peering over a Toyota instruction manual. Professionals in action.

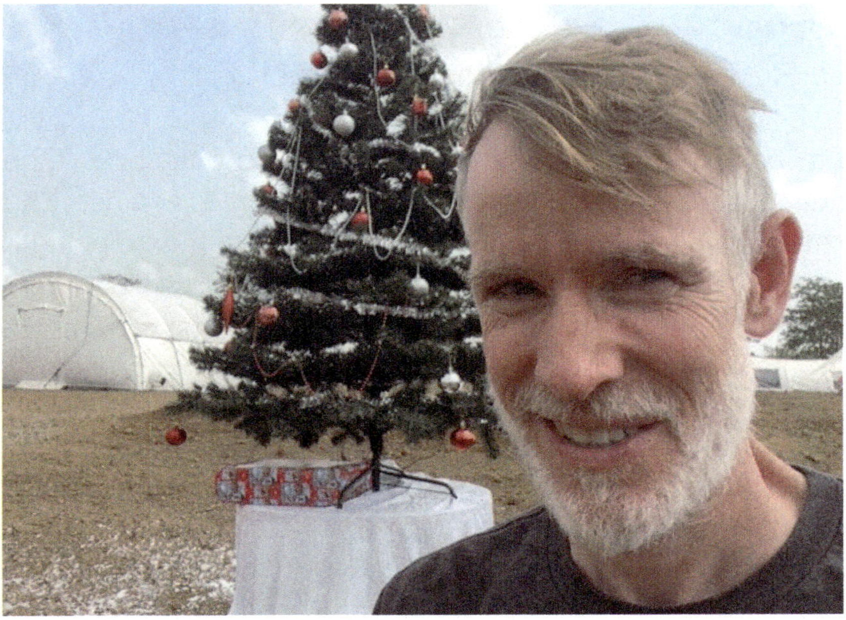

When we get to the next town we are informed that the Paramount Chief has moved once more. He appears to be the Scarlet Pimpernel of Moymaba district. Another ‘couple of miles’ and I am preparing myself for a future lifetime in a wheelchair. We decide the hunt is over and leave the army and police to carry on so we can return to Moyamba before dark.

The news is good on my return. The water is returning and the tankers have arrived. We re-open for business and our first patient quickly arrives. Christmas Eve and I head to the hospital for my festive night on call. A quick photo next to the Norwegian Christmas tree - they tell me it’s one of their finest firs, but I suspect they are lying.

Thursday, 25 December 2014
It's a Red Zone Christmas

It is a red (zone) Christmas for me. The Ebola hospital is quiet but our patients fluctuate wildly in their fight against Ebola, sometimes well enough to get up and walk, but then dipping into semi-consciousness and near moribund states. Ebola is a rolla coasta.
Seven patients and just one death so far since we opened. For Ibrahim there is a suggestion that there might have been other factors beyond Ebola contributing to his death. It was strange how he deteriorated so quickly, and he was complaining of back pain and pain at the back of his head before he lost consciousness. I hear from one of the drivers that he resisted admission when he was first diagnosed, and was beaten badly before he came into hospital. Some elements of the police and the army have a reputation for excessive force. They won't have risked touching him so I wonder if rifle butts or sticks were involved and, with his impaired clotting from the haemorrhagic fever, if he might have had a cerebral bleed. We will never know, as a post mortem is impossible these days but I ask the head of the district Ebola response team to make some discreet enquiries anyway.

The night shift of nurses and watsans have taken to sitting outside the floodlit dressing tent in rows of chairs, watching the entrancing spectacle of relays of teams donning their PPE. The strangeness of our dressing routines, as if dressing for a masked ball, provides an engaging nightly theatre.

I am on call with Chris, a Norwegian paramedic. We join the spectators and sit talking through our Christmas Eve on call.

Many of the watsan are teachers, now unemployed with the closure of all the schools, so they are bright and entertaining with their insight into local life and recent history. They have taken jobs as hygienists; high risk but low paid jobs cleaning up the toxic diarrhoea and vomit on the wards.

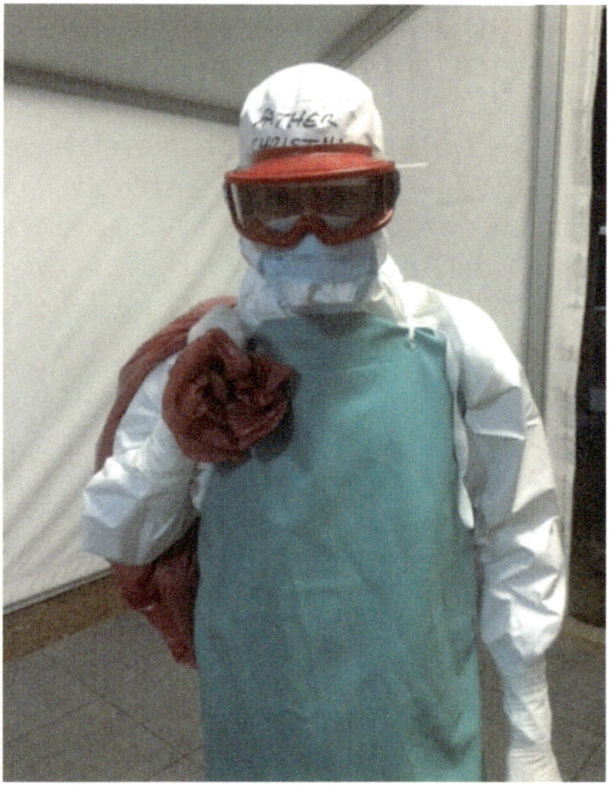

They talk about how Ebola has changed their lives. Christmas used to be a time of great celebration and joyful parties; dancing on the beach until dawn. Now all such gatherings are banned. Christmas has been cancelled. Tomorrow will be another dull day with families and friends isolated from each other by self-imposed quarantine.

They tell us about the devastation caused by the recent civil war. Moyamba was a thriving district capital with running water and electricity but the rebel Westside boys set up camp nearby and would come into town with murderous intent. The rebels smashed everything they found.

As we sit enveloped by the warm African night air, the staff recall their personal experiences of the torture the rebels inflicted. The drugged-up boy soldiers would tease their victims with choices of mutilations: long sleeve, short sleeve or sleeveless depending on where the arm would be cut off with a machete. They describe how they witnessed decapitations of their neighbours; how pregnant women would be cut open on a casual wager over the sex of the baby. How mothers would be forced to laugh while their children were brutally killed.

Mohammed, one of the dressers, tells me with pride how he was a soldier in the Sierra Leonean army, trained by the Scottish light infantry. He was caught in an ambush during the war and tortured and bayoneted. He shows me the scars on his arms and his back, and talks of the scars in his mind that are much slower to heal.

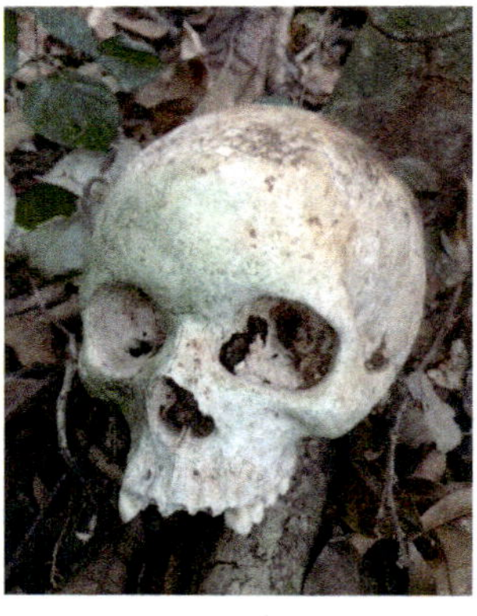

This is such recent trauma, so visible on the bodies and in the minds of Sierra Leoneans. Walking in a forest near the camp at the weekend I had stumbled across a grim reminder of the violence when I almost stepped on a skull. I picked it up with medical curiosity to inspect it for signs of trauma and wondered about the tragic back story. Was it a man or a woman? Had they be hiding in the forest and found or had they been taken there to be executed? I dug a shallow grave to bring some peace and rest to this lost soul.

So much destruction and cruelty in such recent history. The seeds of the Ebola and cholera epidemics in the country are a legacy of this war. The wanton destruction of infrastructure - water supplies, electricity, sewage systems - and the failure to repair this in the subsequent peace.

As the early hours of the morning seep in through the open tent Chris takes pity on the staff and for some reason decides that an introduction to Norwegian music might be exactly what they need to soothe their mental wounds. I am overcome with a sudden urge to stick a blanket over my head and to try to sleep.

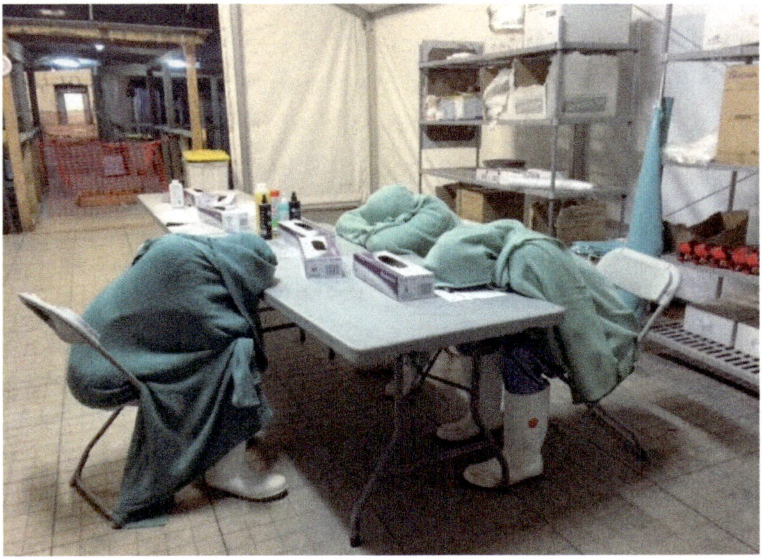

Friday, 26 December 2014
Close to Victory: The Lions on the Mountain

Christmas Day passes uneventfully. We are reminded at the morning Command and Control meeting that Ebola does not take a holiday, although in Moyamba apparently it does. The house to house searching prior to Christmas identified no cases. Numbers of referrals remain low. All the evidence points to a petering out of the epidemic outside Freetown. This is great news, though having just set up a 100 bed treatment centre, I have to suppress my evil-villain-with-a-hand-wringing-demonic-laugh desire for more Ebola. Having seen the suffering it causes, I am of course delighted. This is a great festive gift of life.

I am coming to the end of my trip. The NGOs call these international attachments missions - an odd reclamation of an old word for religious colonisation. The entire international aid community appears to have descended on this country and I wonder what the nationals think about this new colonial invasion, with good intentions in place of guns and germs.

I am familiar with the international aid community in my previous global health work, but I have never experienced such a dense concentration. They are easy enough to spot in Sierra Leone - as anyone who is white is involved in the Ebola response. The business people left months ago and will return slowly and cautiously to make money when they get a cast iron all clear guarantee.

I have learnt much on my mission. Most of all I have learnt that this war on Ebola has been fought by Africans and that the blood that has been shed is African blood. We have arrived late into this battle, and ended up as stretcher bearers rather than fighters. The real heroes of this emergency are the Sierra Leonean health care workers who have stood bravely on the front line while we have watched from a safe distance, frozen by caution and fear.

When the first cases of Ebola were reported in May 2014 the health care system retaliated with beautifully simple, but remarkably effective, designs to protect themselves and their patients. These early Heath Robinson Ebola units have been the frontier forts defending communities against the relentless attacks from Ebola.

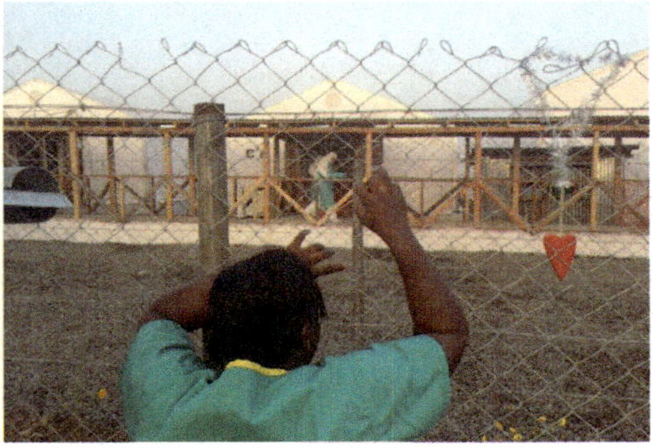

The West's response was too late to the starting line and probably over-engineered at the finish. Our Ebola Treatment Centres are undoubtedly too big and too clever. However, when they were commissioned in September the predictions for Ebola were 1.4 million casualties by January, so it would have been a brave decision back then to build fewer beds. And of course the Centres are just one link in our chain of support. We have worked hard to support the behavioural change and social mobilisation programmes, safe burials, surveillance and logistics.

I have learnt much about the challenges of complex international collaborations in an emergency setting. We have made many mistakes in this response. I am sure lessons will be carefully documented, quietly forgotten and then inevitably repeated. These are such simple, common-sense lessons: good leadership; clear organisational structures and boundaries; listening to the staff on the front line; harnessing their talent and creativity; managing with a light touch and positive stroking. These lessons are as true for an international emergency as for an NHS hospital.

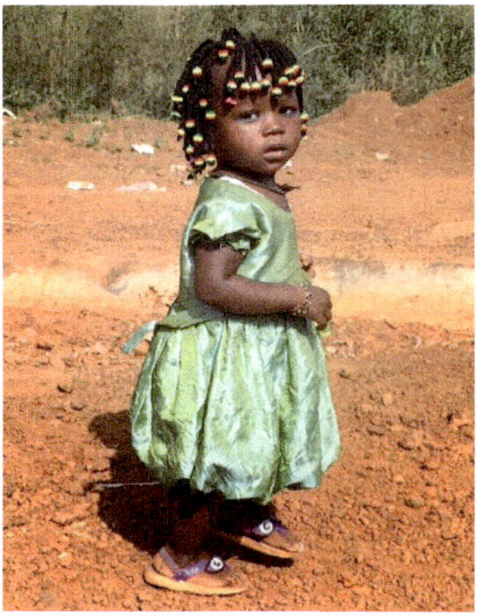

There is an old African proverb: if you want to go fast then go alone; if you want to go far then go together. We have gone fast and far in these past few weeks. Now it is time for me to go home.

I am reticent about returning to my daily routines in the UK. I love my job but I know it will be difficult to sit through the next committee meeting with the same level of engagement as before. I miss my wife and family, but I am already feeling choked about not being able to touch and hug them as I step through the door after 6 weeks away.

I have been deeply touched with the kindness and support I have received since I have been here. I am just a fleeting shadow, an amanuensis recording a remarkable tale of one country's struggle against a devastating and malevolent foe. All praise, respect, admiration and acclaim goes to the people of Sierra Leone who have suffered, rallied and are now close to victory. Lions on the mountain.

Tuesday, 30 December 2014
Take me home, country road, West Moyamba

I had intended the previous diary entry to be my final one. Knowing when to stop is a judgement call, but my last day in Moyamba felt like an appropriate time. Harping on about the cold and consumerism on return is a sure way to generate stifled yawns.

However, two subsequent events have prompted me to continue for a little while longer. Two events that take me from joy to fear on this emotionally labile Ebola journey.

There was much happiness on my last morning in Moyamba with the announcement of our first survivor. Saffie was the older women admitted on our first day, with her age, and her poor clinical state on admission, her chances of survival seemed low. Against considerable odds she clung on to life and escaped the dark stormy crossing of her illness. She would rally and then fade and we would fear the worst as she dropped back into semi-consciousness. One week to the day after we opened our Ebola centre she was well enough to consider a blood test. The result was returned the next morning and I could not have wished for a better farewell gift, a wonderful souvenir to cherish.

There are two exits from the red zone. The first is the mortuary exit, and half our patients will pass through this door on their way to safe burial. The second is the 'happy door' with a shower of chlorinated water and then the sweet freedom of the green zone. Saffie exited through the happy door to pick up her life once more. She will continue to face adversity as she tries to integrate back into her village. Ebola survivors are stigmatised and shunned. Their community will fear them as carriers and be suspicious of their return. Everything she owns will be burnt (clothes, blankets, mattresses) or decontaminated, in a scorched earth approach to Ebola eradication. But she is alive, and the whole team is buzzing with excitement. This is what we have come here for: curing Ebola, one patient at a time.

I said my farewells and hit the Moyamba road back towards Freetown and the airport five hours away. There, I was reunited with my NHS colleagues from Kerrytown and Port Loko. The team who had been sent to Emergency in Laka had ended up resigning over ethical concerns about the drugs and interventional approach being used there. They had relocated to Kerrytown where they had settled well and felt they had been able to make a valuable contribution. The Port Loko team had been slow to open but had got there in the end, with a similar sense of accomplishment. Some were hoping to return, everyone was excited about going home.

Our Casablanca flight left a deserted Freetown airport at 02.30 and landed four sleepy hours later. We were greeted by men in biohazard suits shouting 'stand back' to us as we queued up for an infrared body scan. Then on to Heathrow where we had a more measured welcome from Public Health England. There was a frisson of excitement in Border Control as 30 high risk Ebola contacts joined the queues for passport checks.

Then, in small groups, we were whisked away for health checks and to have our temperature measured. It was all rather chaotic and disorganised, with growing frustration amongst the volunteers who were exhausted and just wanted to get home, but the public health team did their best to remain calm and

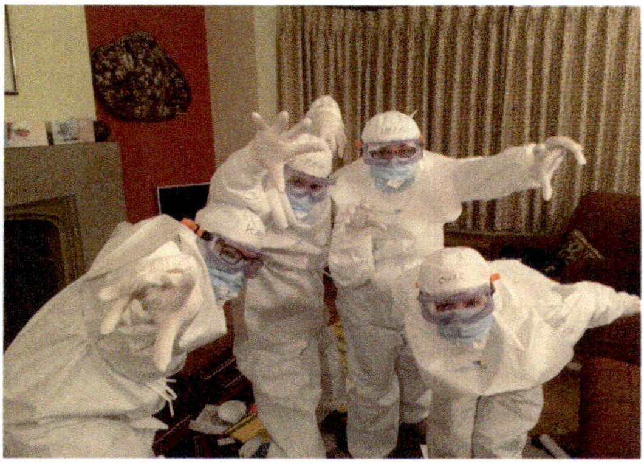

collected doling out a home-coming gift of biohazard bags, gloves, disinfectant and plastic scoops for any vomit and diarrhoea we may have.

Then home and a wonderful daddy, my daddy welcome from my family at the station in the spirit of the Railway Children. Cautious no-skin-contact hugs and a joyful home reunion.

I have missed Christmas and there was not a huge selection of gifts in Moyamba, so I had smuggled back four sets of PPE for their belated Christmas presents. The early hours of the morning found us rehearsing donning and doffing routines and then dancing to ABBA in full PPE. It was all a bit surreal

One of my daughters gives up her bedroom for my one degree of separation, but by the following afternoon I am becoming more laissez faire over my intended self-imposed isolation. As we sit down in high spirits for our family Christmas dinner in the evening, my daughter reads out from her phone that there has been a case of Ebola in Glasgow. Breaking news throws out small clues until it is clear who the individual is: Pauline Cafferkey, one of the Save the Children nurses, who was transferred to a high-level isolation unit at the Royal Free for a long and grueling rcovery.

What an awful shock. I am worried for her - how terrifying it must be to wake up with a fever, knowing the consequences. Then the ambulance convoy and isolation pod flight to London. All alone with no one to hold your hand.

I am also worried for myself and my family. I have become blasé about the risk of infection during my stay in Sierra Leone. Now I am in my safe European home and already feel that I am immune, although I still have nearly three weeks before I am released from my quarantine parole. This case brings the risk starkly home to me and planned trips to the cinema, a rapid return to work and perhaps even a New Year's Eve get-together are all quickly postponed. I distribute my returned stock of alcohol gel bottles to my family and we agree to revert to a no-touch policy. The risk of transmission is negligible but they will be the ones most at risk if I do develop symptoms, so it's important we take precautions. They are alarmed but sensible; it is the wider reception of the news that worried me. A case of Ebola in the first wave of returning NHS volunteers will amplify fear and prejudice. The scaremongering newspaper headlines are already screaming out.

Public Health England quickly establishes contact with me for daily monitoring. I will phone in my temperatures twice a day and notify them immediately if I develop any symptoms. They are helpful and supportive and it is comforting to know they are with me. My wife suggests I shave my beard to be less identifiable in public when we go out. Maybe some plastic surgery, though I am banned from any interventional procedures for now.

Wednesday, 31 December 2014
Root Cause Analysis

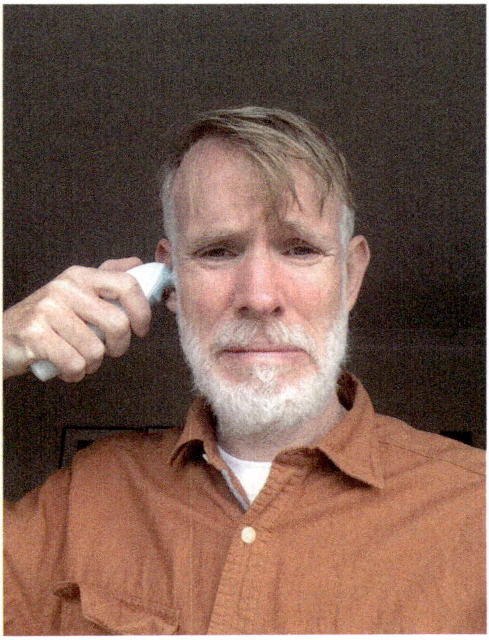

My twice daily temperature checks have taken on a new urgency. I have been half-hearted about these checks, and normalised to the interminable fever checks in Sierra Leone. The news about my colleague changes this and I am now nervous every time I take out the thermometer. Is there such a thing as 'white coat' fever?

Public Health England have issued us with high quality aural thermometers. The action of putting this to my ear is similar to that of holding a gun to the side of my head, and the implications of the reading when I press the trigger generates a feeling of Russian roulette. My Christmas charade is a twice daily recreation of The Deer Hunter.

I have had a lot of requests for interviews from the media but I will turn them all down as I have nothing useful to contribute to what is a very private tragedy. Journalists, for the most part, do a tough, poorly paid job and play a powerful role in informing society. Good relationships with them are crucial to keep up the level of public awareness about the Ebola emergency, and also to explain how we are using tax payers money to save lives.

However, my colleague's Ebola infection, like all critical illness, is a personal concern. She asked for privacy, and we should respect this, although inevitably, within a few hours of the news breaking, her personal details are all over the papers.

There is discontent within my NHS cohort of returnees about some of our number wading in to provide ill-informed media commentaries, feeding the hyperbole and speculation about Ebola. There are suggestions that the PHE screening at Heathrow was inadequate, but this is probably unfair and informed by hindsight. Fever screening was negative for all of us and so there was no indication for further action. The following morning it was positive for my colleague, so she immediately contacted our helpline. This is how screening works: when you get a positive result you take action. Until then you remain calm. The alternative would have been to keep us all in a quarantine tent for 21 days just to be sure none of us develop a fever. Any review of our Heathrow screening is best left to the professionals at Public Health England rather than unqualified bystanders.

There is also much poorly informed speculation about how my colleague was exposed. Our personal protection is robust, and we report any breaches that might occur, but only when we notice them. When MSF investigated the 26 or so staff from their centre in Bo who had been infected, they found that the source was usually in the community - a friend or neighbour with Ebola who had informally asked for medical help.

One major gap in our Ebola response is the lack of systematic root cause analysis of these safety alerts. Determining the contributory factors is essential to improving the safety for staff, but the myriad of agencies involved in providing care hinders a standardised and robust approach. I was told that CDC was going to take oversight, but I have not seen any reports as yet, and with the continuing notifications of national and international health care workers, this review and learning should be a top priority.

Meanwhile Chris emails me from Moyamba with details of his night on call - illustrating the chaotic nature of life in an Ebola hospital

Hi John

Yesterday evening it was announced at the Command and Control meeting that 4 patients were coming up from Ribbi as Ebola suspects. I phoned the duty doctor at the centre that we had four on the way but no ETA

By 7pm nobody had arrived and so I phoned Alfred to ask where the patients were. He told me that they were 'on their way'.

8pm I phoned again. They were at the Holding Centre. Alfred had diverted them there as their paperwork was not complete and he said he would transfer them in the morning
A full team of staff had been on stand-by at the ETC, and I insisted that the patients be transferred at once. He agreed.

He then phoned back half an hour later to say that the driver refused to drive after dark.
I contacted Capt F and told him that this was not satisfactory and that we would take the patients now or send our own ambulance to fetch them

At 10 pm SEVEN patients arrived in one ambulance including one sick three year old whose mother had died of Ebola and whose healthy sister had been left behind at the Holding Centre as they could not pack any more people into the ambulance. I sent the ambulance back to get the sister to look after the child so now we had eight admissions. the patients being admitted told me that there were still SIX more patients in the Holding Centre.

We finished admitting at 1am. So we now have eight new suspect patients and probably six more in the Holding Centre. Of the eight patients, three are pretty ill probably look like Ebola. So we have three probables, plus five contaminated suspects, and we have to make a decision about the other six patients this morning.

Chris

Thursday, 1 January 2015
A Hermit's New Year's Eve

A hermit's New Year's Eve for me. My risk of transmission to others is minimal, but in view of the media frenzy I think it best for me to avoid crowded indoor venues. I could get used to this anti-social way of life.

I have been picking up my life and venturing out for walks and to the shops. When I meet people who I know they instinctively put out their hand to welcome me. I feel like Anton Ferdinand meeting John Terry as I politely snub them. I am more conscious than ever about skin contact. I also have this strange sense of

Ebola paranoia that everyone is staring at me. Maybe it's the flashing reindeer antlers I am wearing on my head.

At 9pm on New Year's Eve a special delivery arrived from Public Health England - more thermometers, disinfectant, gloves and biohazard bags for vomit. Maybe they are anticipating the outcome of my daughters' late night celebrations.

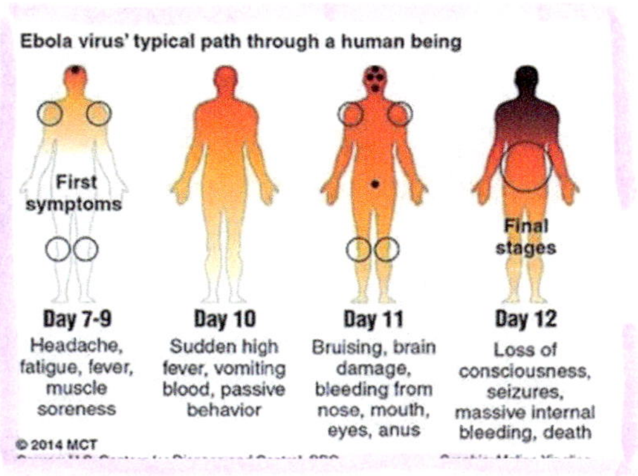
Ebola virus' typical path through a human being
First symptoms
Final stages
Day 7-9
Headache, fatigue, fever, muscle soreness
Day 10
Sudden high fever, vomiting blood, passive behavior
Day 11
Bruising, brain damage, bleeding from nose, mouth, eyes, anus
Day 12
Loss of consciousness, seizures, massive internal bleeding, death
© 2014 MCT

My twice daily temperatures provide traction through the day. I have that natural optimism bias that I will be fine, based on hope rather than reason. As no one is quite sure how other health care workers are getting infected, there remains the real possibility that I may be harbouring an early infection. Incubation is up to 21 days, but usually between 7-9 days. I am now 7 days post-exposure, so approaching my day of reckoning. I have been using the chart below to plan the remainder of our festive celebrations. I have suggested a day in front of the telly for Day 12.

My main worry is not Ebola, but the risk of getting a fever from another cause - the coughs and colds that are going around at this time of year. At any other time this would mean a Lemsip and an early night. These days it will mean a convoy of ambulances and police cars to my nearest specialist centre in Sheffield.

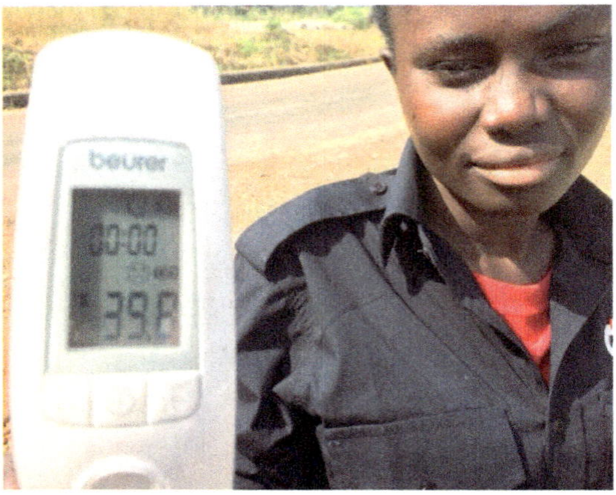

Fevers in Sierra Leone led to isolation at home until it settled. I did get a few scares at the fever security checks. 'Oh oh spaghettio' I tweeted the photo below. My wife did not see the funny side. The guards still let me through. 40 degrees was the usual cut off in Sierra Leone, sometimes even 41. In the UK the cut off is currently 37.5. In Belgium and Australia it is 38. In India it is 38.3. In Spain and the US it is 38.6. I might have to emigrate depending on what threshold I can meet.

Sunday 4 January 2015

Rather predictably I have developed a fever. Yesterday was spent nursing prodromal, flu-like symptoms – sore throat, headache and generally feeling poorly. It is probably just a seasonal winter virus but the big fear, particularly after Pauline's diagnosis, is that it could be Ebola.

I notify my local public health minder who explains that they will have to send out a Hazmat team – paramedics and police all dressed in full PPE to pick take me to nearest Ebola containment unit in Leeds. I feel an acute suburban embarrassment of 'what will the neighbours think?' as blue light emergency vehicles pile up outside the house. "Can't I just drive to the hospital?" I ask.

“Well, it is against guidance, and if you do it is without me knowledge, but if you want to then I will arrange for the Infectious Disease team to meet you there’ he helpfully offers.

I take the 15 year old Renault Clio on the basis that if I have Ebola, and the car needs to be burnt then it will be no big loss. “Wipe all the surface down!” is my parting cry as I set off. “Horse. Bolted” my daughter astutely replies “If you’ve got Ebola then we all have”.

I arrive at St James Hospital in Leeds on a quiet Sunday morning and park at the back at a pre-arranged spot. Two Infectious Disease nurses provide a surreal welcoming party, shepherding me in through the delivery entrance.

On the ward I am shown my own secure private room with a decontamination area outside, and settle down to await the medics. Five minutes later I hear the sound of the medical team attempting to don PPE for the first time. “Where does this go?” “How do I put this on?” “What on earth is this?”. Part of me wants to go out and help them, but that might defeat the object of my isolation.

Half an hour later and my bloods have been sent to Porton Down for testing, and I begin a nervous 24 hour wait. After all the news frenzy over Pauline Cafferkey, rather perversely I was more worried about the media attention from a diagnosis of Ebola than the actual virus. Conscious that if I did have Ebola then the press would pick one of the worst photos of me (so many to choose from!) and reprint this ad nauseam, I quit social media (for a while…).

The next day the results came back and and I breathed a deep sigh of relief as I was cleared for discharge.

****

Returning back to civilian life was a relief. There was a bit of anxiety in the first few days from some of my colleagues about the risk of catching Ebola from me. Even my wife in Leeds came up against a bit of prejudice by association. However life quickly returned to welcome normality and I jumped back on my Bradford horse and picked up the reins.

In May 2015 I was invited to a dinner hosted by Richard Rogers at the House of Lords for the syndicate of 30 global Presidents of the Medicins du Monde/Doctors of the World (a bit like SPECTRE, but for good) and asked to give a speech to a) highlight the on-going health emergency in Sierra Leone and b) make a shameless pitch to Lord Rogers to come and redesign my kitchen. The first part went down well, but Lord Rogers remained impassive about the second. In rejection I turned to the leading kitchen architect partnership of Ikea, Ikea and Allenkey.

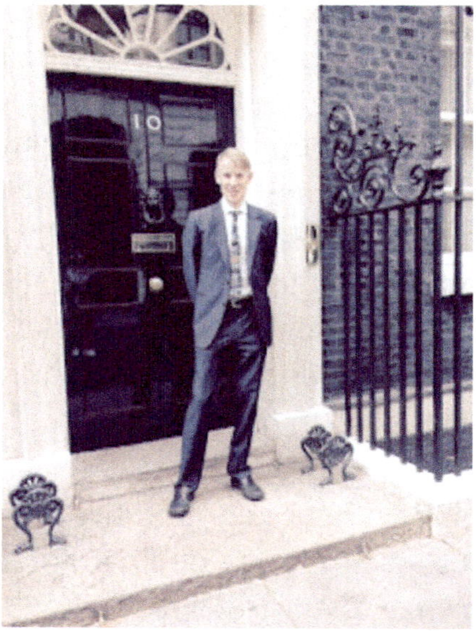

In July I was invited to Downing Street on behalf of Doctors of the World to be awarded the Ebola medal ("sounds dangerous" my daughter mused). As a male I do suffer from a moderately severe form of the Y-chromosomal disorder imposter syndrome, but never have I felt it so acutely as on this occasion. I met up with some of my NHS and DFID colleagues from the mission as well as Dave Cameron (pompous), Jeremy Hunt (creepy), Michael Fallon ('hello chaps!" (yes, really)) and Justine Greening (normal human being – what is she doing in the cabinet). Also a great meeting with Peter Piot from the LSHTM who was one of the first doctors to manage Ebola in the very first outbreak in 1976. He described how they coped with very limited resources, borrowing the motorcycle goggles of the local missionary to protect his eyes and Marigold gloves as PPE.

One Year On: return to Moyamba

Friday, 13 November 2015
A happy Ebola-versary

One year ago after I travelled to Sierra Leone with Doctors of the World to help set up and run an Ebola Treatment Centre in Moyamba. Last Saturday Sierra Leone was declared Ebola-free. What a time for joy and celebration after such an age of suffering and fear. Bye bye Ebola.

Over the last few months I have been working with my public health colleagues on a detailed health needs assessment and review of health systems. We found a breakdown in trust between communities and health services, significant reductions in health service use, increasing mortality and falling immunisation rates. All the attention and focus on Ebola, loss of clinical staff from the disease and fear about health centres being 'plague centres' has created a second public health emergency.

Today I am heading back. My mission for DOTW for the next two weeks is two-fold 1) to work with the district health team to strengthen health systems and surveillance 2) to liaise with international government donors and the WHO to explore how NGOs can help support the fragile health service. In addition I will be linking up with the Public Health England team in Freetown to explore joint working, doing some epidemiological work about the clinical sequelae of Ebola and observing the decommissioning of the Moyamba Ebola Treatment Centre.

The BBC are keen on another Radio 4 programme (budgets are tight and my services are free) – a Christmas show, though not very Morecambe and Wise. So on Wednesday I had a trip to Broadcasting House to meet the documentary team and my producer Sue. There I get taken down to the basement to meet the BBC 'Q' (disappointingly named Adam) and get fitted out with a bewildering array of microphones and recording devices. Sue was planning to come with me but at the last minute has changed her mind and instead was flown off to the furthest geographical point from Sierra Leone, with supportive advice "it's probably all safe now" ringing in my ears.

It will be interesting to see how society has changed as the curtain of death has been raised. Will people be touching each other? Are the army checkpoints still in place? How are the survivors coping? What has happened to the ETC in Moyamba? Let's see how I get on.

Monday, 16 November 2015
Saturday

I touchdown in Paris and connect to my Freetown flight a few hours after l"horreur of the Islamist terrorist attacks in the city. Charles de Gaulle airport carries on its global churn of humanity as though nothing has happened. I want to hug the cabin staff and show some humanity, but they meet and greet the passengers with automatic professionalism, as though nothing has happened. Last year the plane to Freetown was filled almost completely with white Europeans - international aid workers rushing to the front line. This time the plane is filled with black Africans - normal service has been resumed.

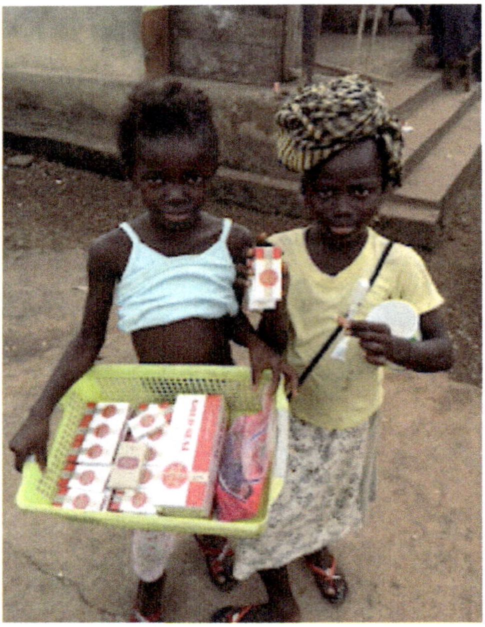

I disembark into moonlit heat of Lungi airport and ride the wave of passengers surging over the tidal defences of bureaucracy. Boarding cards please! (I left mine on the plane thinking "Ronseal" but have no intention of going back to get it so use the momentum of those behind crying "forward!" to duck past). Yellow cards please! (these might be yellow fever certificates, but I don't have one of these either so seize a moment of distraction to dive past this one), a hand washing station with an obligatory squirt of alcohol gel. Then the unavoidable visa checks, border checks, health checks and finally the temperature checks. Everyone's temperature is raised by this stage, but fortunately the cheap Chinese infrared thermometers fail to register it.

It was a strange relief to escape into the organised chaos of bus and boat transfers to Freetown where everyone is trying to make a buck. Sierra Leone is the 184th poorest country in the world (there are only 187 countries, so I am hoping for some regression to the mean this year) and the sense of desperation for those at the bottom, hawking tickets or drinks or foreign exchange is heart-breaking. I thank the God of DNA Migration that my children will never have to fight for the basic Maslow-vian needs, though another four years of the Tories and they may yet be flogging dusty bottles of Coke outside Heathrow.

Sunday

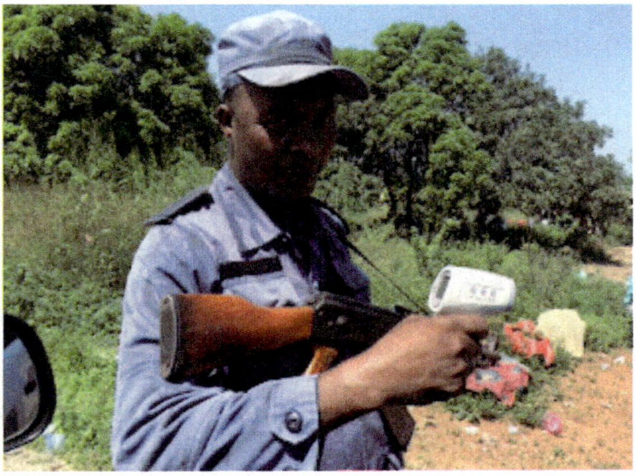

An overnight stay at the DOTW office where there is no food. I am starving. In Africa. The irony. Then it's an early start for the long journey back to Moyamba. The last time I made this journey the country was at peak-Ebola. The roads were empty from the travel bans. The market places deserted from the prohibition on public gatherings. Hoardings glared down from the road-sides with their messages of death. Army checkpoints enforced sombre fever checks with monotonous regularity.

What a difference a year makes. The journey could not have been more dissimilar. The roads are full of hustle and bustle. Pop-up shops and market stalls have returned with their life-blood of daily trade. Groups assemble at in the shade of trees and corrugated metal shelters, talking and laughing, holding hands. I glimpse a snatched kiss and consider its poignancy as I speed through the lush and verdant countryside. This is a country that has been under a wicked Ebola queen's curse. A sleeping beauty awoken by a symbolic kiss.

The occasional army checkpoint survives but the mood is light and carefree. I ask a soldier why he is still checking my temperature now that Ebola has gone. He tells me that there is still a 90 day period of surveillance, but his half-hearted effort suggests this is more of a fading habit than serious intent. He waves us on nonchalantly, thermometer in one hand, AK47 in the other.

The contrast from last year is unsettling. Everything is so normal I feel as though I may have dreamt Ebola. I marvel at the resilience of humankind.

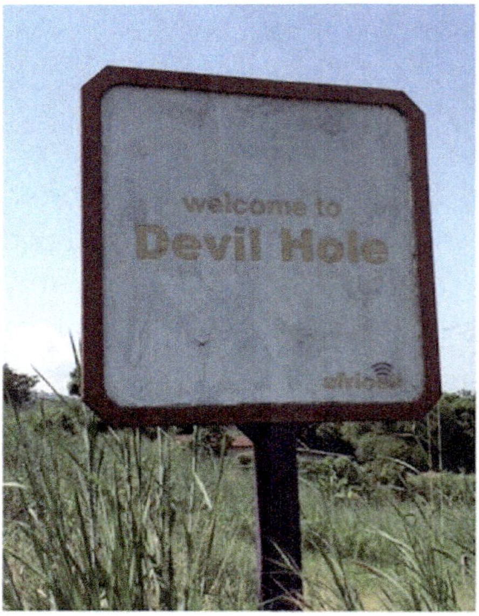
welcome to
Devil Hole

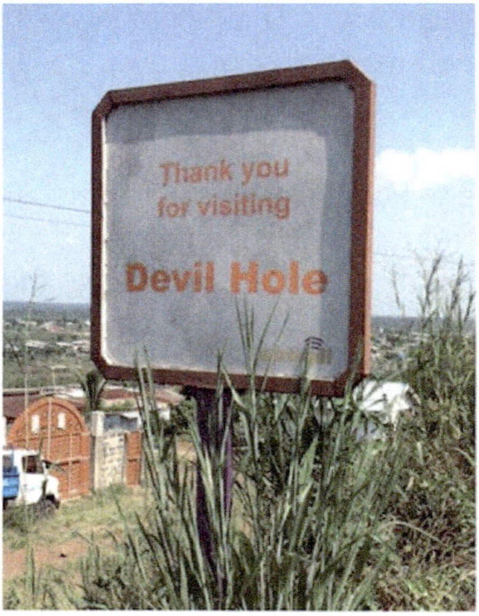
Thank you
for visiting
Devil Hole

The road has deteriorated significantly over the last year. A metaphor for the country's economy. We drive past familiar towns, taking a break in one called "Devil's Hole". Last year this felt like nominative determinism. Now I think the town council should give serious thought to rebranding if they are going to seek inward investment.

At a petrol station further on I spot a Landcruiser with "Teenage Pregnancy Reduction Project" on its doors and wander over to find out more. Maude Peacock is President of the Women's Forum in Sierra Leone and describes with vim and passion the work they are doing to help teenage girls - both during the war and then the Ebola epidemic. The school closures were the "Devil's workshop" for the current epidemic of teenage pregnancies. I wonder if the Devils Hole town council should consider bidding to host it.

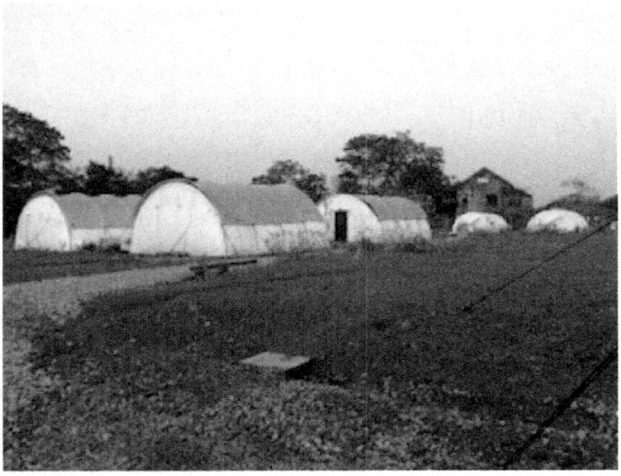

The Norwegian base camp in Moyamba looks tired and dirty. There are only a dozen staff left, a ragbag of logisticians, water and sanitation (watsans) and a doctor and nurse who have been doing ongoing training for local health clinics. A mixture of Spanish, French, Italian and Lebanese. I am the only Brit, though strictly speaking I am travelling on an Irish passport (useful for trips to Pakistan/Iran to avoid being chained to a radiator, and to Ebola nations when you want to avoid rejection at border controls - everyone should have one - let's do a deal with Eire) and quickly fail the Tebbit test by not knowing about the big game tomorrow.

The camp is being rapidly dismantled and the tents sent back to DFID. With a limited stock of alternative accommodation I fear I may end up back in the derelict stadium. But there is food and I gorge.

Tuesday, 17 November 2015
How to dismantle an Ebola bomb

I am strangely nervous about returning to the ETC on my pilgrimage to Moyamba, coming back to the battlefield one year on, after the war has been won.

The last patient was discharged a couple of months ago, and I half expect a deserted facility so am surprised by the level of activity I find. Groups of staff in surgical scrubs are busy at work decontaminating and dismantling the Centre. They greet me with a touching joy and warmth.

I move from group to group exchanging greetings and news. The site is still a high risk centre for Ebola contamination, but after a year of avoiding body contact everyone is demob happy and we shake hands and hug each other for the first time ever, savouring this forbidden fruit of touch. We exchange stories about the early days of the ETC - from recruitment and training to our first nervous shifts in the red zone. Old soldiers recounting stories from the war.

There is great happiness about the end of Ebola, but a scratch beneath the surface and I find sadness and worry about the impending loss of their jobs. They were ready to take their chance with the acute threat of Ebola, but unemployment is the long term condition that they fear the most. There are no jobs in Moyamba and they face a bleak future.

There are only two nurses left working at the ETC. Janet and Rose welcome me with screams. Happy screams I am relieved to find. Janet was working with me when we admitted our first ever Ebola patients and tells me about two of our early survivors - Isatu and Safi. Both are back to good health. Isatu is pregnant now - new life from near death.

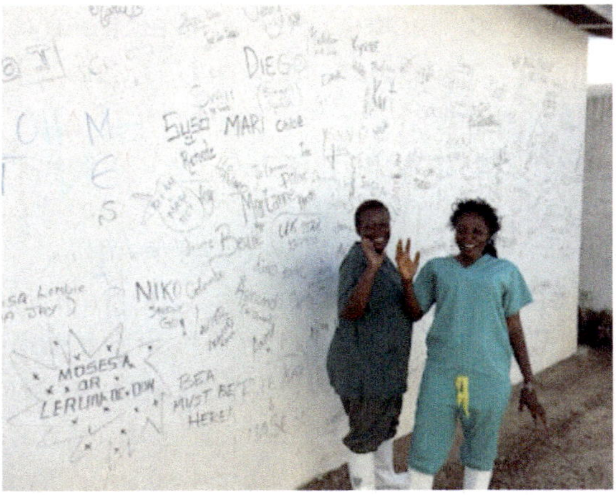

But it is their last day and tomorrow they too are out of work and demoralised. The health service has too little money to recruit their precious talent. The contrast is unsettling. I go out for a few weeks and get feted with undeserved glory. They put their lives at risk for the entire epidemic and get made redundant. Taking the example from Sonny Bill Williams I promise to send Janet my Ebola medal.

They are proud of their contribution to stopping the epidemic. Proud also that had no Ebola casualties in the workforce. A safe centre for its staff and its patients and one of the few ETCs to be able to make this claim. I take a final picture of them outside the nurses station, now covered with farewell graffiti like a school-leavers shirt.

How to dismantle a toxic Ebola hospital: a quick and easy recipe

Ingredients

1. Tents. The tents have plastic walls and can be safely decontaminated with by spraying high strength chlorine solution. The roof is a challenge as its five metres high.
2. Equipment. Mattresses, plastic buckets and metal trolleys are asked in soap and then sprayed in chlorine. These will be donated to the local community.
3. Pipes and taps. The 0.5% chlorine has eroded all the metal pipes. No one is confident that rust and erosion can be properly cleaned from Ebola so, these will be destroyed.
4. Wood. The wooden roofs and walkways, so beautifully constructed by the Royal Engineers from the finest African hardwood also have to be destroyed. WHO have decreed that as wood is porous and we know so little about how the virus can survive, no risk can be taken. Six tons of wooden craftsmanship have been dismantled and burnt in giant pits.

Instructions

1. Don full personal protective equipment (PPE) and enter the red zone.
2. Soap down and spray with chlorine every surface making sure not to miss a single spot.
3. Dismantle the wooden corridors bolt by bolt, nail by nail (don't get a nail-stick injury!), timber by timber.
4. The temperature in your PPE will rise to over 50 degrees. The sweat will soak your mask and give the sensation of drowning while you are undertaking a heavy labouring job, so no more than 20 minutes attacks on the structure before you head for the doffing area.

5. Repeat for two months

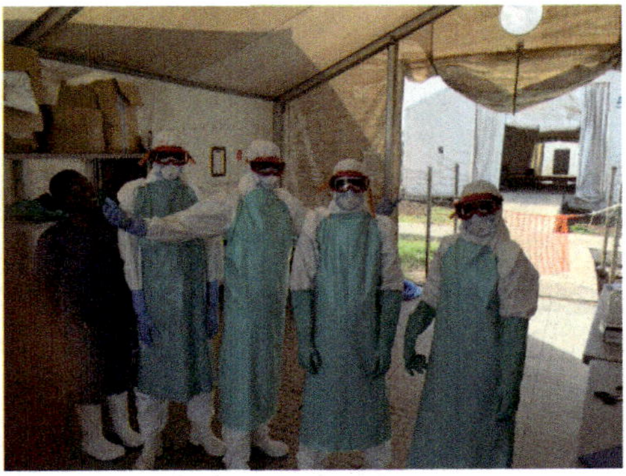

The chef for this main course is Xavier, a Spanish chemical and biological decontamination engineer who has had to organise a complex rotating system of dismantlers to manage the task.

Just sitting in the shade is exhausting in the heat and humidity and I thought that the clinical work in PPE was endurance-testing. Watching the watsans dressed in full PPE doing heavy construction work filled me with awe.

Wednesday, 18 November 2015
'Bradford's latest weekly notification report....'

There is a calm efficiency to the decline and fall of the Ebola Treatment Centre. The opening was a madness of urgency and rush. Today the international staff sit relaxed in front of laptops showing spreadsheets of logistics and the watsans continue their slow but methodical dismantling.

Was it all worth it? The final score for Ebola in Sierra Leone was 14,089 cases, 10,134 survivors and 3,955 deaths. A survival rate which looks a healthy 72% is flattered by a reporting bias. All the survivors will have been identified, but many of the deaths will have been missed in the community. A good illustration of this can be found in the health workers. These are much more likely to have been picked up and reported, and out of the 307 cases only 86 survived - an identical rate of 72%, but this time flipped from a survival rate to a mortality rate.

My arrival in the country last November coincided with the peak in reporting in the country, and my departure with a reassuring trough. While it is tempting to claim causal attribution, this may be pushing the interpretation of the evidence (though I will include this on my CV).

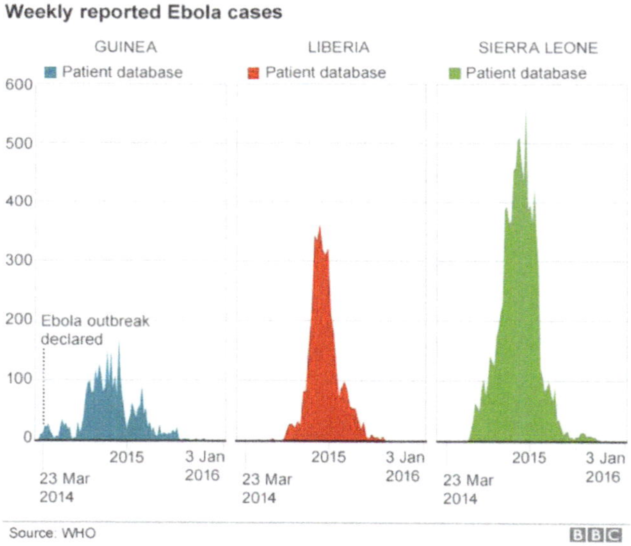

A recent paper in the Proceedings of the National Academy of Sciences attempted to model what the impact was. The authors estimated that the opening of the 12 Ebola Treatment Centres saved 57,000 lives - an impressive result in today's underwhelming medical world. I felt at the time that we could have arrived on the scene earlier. The authors look at this too and estimate that an extra 12,000 lives would have been saved if the ETCs had opened a month earlier. Not as many as I expected.

There has been an opportunity cost to all this frenzied activity. Immunisation rates have fallen as families stay away from health centres. Family planning services have been shunned and other infectious diseases neglected. The longer term consequences of this remain uncertain, but the urgency to rebuilding the health service is clear.

The first step for this rebuilding is to re-establish the trust of the community in their health services - a tricky thing to engineer and something that will come naturally with time as the epidemic recedes. The MDM/DOTW team in Moyamba are working with partners to strengthen clean water supplies and hand washing - starting with all the schools in the district. Training of the community health workers comes next - better identification, reporting and referral of all infectious diseases. I attend one of the local workshops where the district health team go through the list of 47 tropical diseases that pose an everyday threat to the community. While some are exotic (Monkey Pox. Chiunkunya. Dracunculiasis) others are routine (measles, cholera) and as always malaria remains the top assassin.

I sit down with the local surveillance team reviewing their reports and systems. One of the key achievements since I was last here is setting up a 'closed user group' mobile phone system which enables the surveillance officers to communicate effectively with the 100 district health units. I check out Bradford's late report which highlights the ongoing threat from malaria.

One of my goals is to explore how we can strengthen the local health system. It feels a bit too centralised and top down - national guidelines via WHO and the ministry pouring out from

Freetown onto a demotivated and demoralised workforce. It is a similar problem in the UK but at least we have the insight to recognise that implementation and improvement need a more grass roots approach: understanding the local context, good leadership, ownership, understanding the facilitators and barriers to change, behavioural change approaches and effective implementation strategies. The ETC remains the focus for everyone's attention in Moyamba, but it is irrelevant now, and our attention should be on the wider health system. Tomorrow I will head out to some of the rural clinics to find out what is happening in the field.

Thursday, 19 November 2015
Camp life

The Norwegian base camp is oddly comforting - I think I may have become institutionalised to communal tent-living with its nocturnal chorus of sighs and snores. However it is rapidly coming down around me and I fear I will be soon homeless. Please don't send me back to the abandoned stadium.

The atmosphere has changed completely since last year. The Norwegian military team did a great job in setting it all up in adverse conditions and looking after us with warm Nordic hospitality, but it was a bit rule-bound and Ebola-paranoid. Now the camp is run by an old Africa-hand Italian who is much more laid back. The atmosphere is more mooching than military, and beer is back on the menu.

The camp apartheid has gone with the lifting of bans on nationals in the camp and it feels much more integrated. Local people have replaced the Norwegians working in the camp and are providing the catering - local flavours and foods (well, fried chicken and rice every night) rather than fish flown in from Oslo.

The Wi-Fi has improved dramatically and there are fewer people to drain it with their devices so I don't have to go begging for internet. Last night the generator failed so we have no power or water and we are all a bit smelly, hungry and Wi-Fi-deprived today. There is the option of the happy shower at the ETC, the one survivors took before they left the red zone, but it's heavily chlorinated so there are few takers.

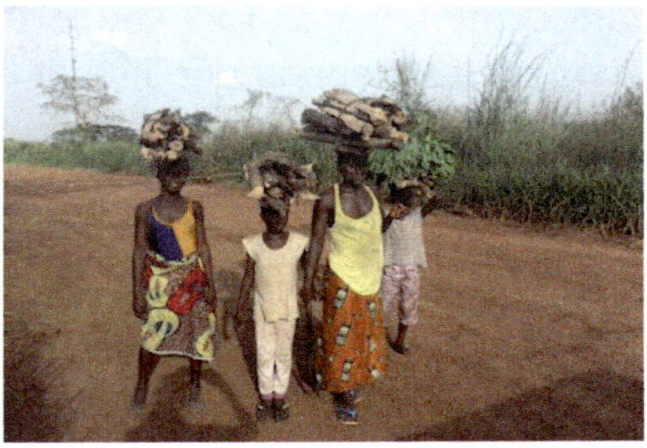

Our polyglot, Babelian community is small and strangely disconnected, thrown together from different countries and different teams - tribal by permutation. The newbies sporting branded NGO T-shirts while the old pros lounge around in faded designer fashion. There is a preponderance of young Mediterranean men with beards who look unnervingly similar and disconcertingly handsome (all you single ladies - think about Moyamba rather than match.com; all you hen parties - give York a break!).

They fill the nocturnal gatherings exchanging stories of near-death experiences from tours in Afghanistan, Somalia, Sudan, CAR. It is an ephemeral life that they live - going from one mission to the next. The balance between their passion to make a difference to the world and keeping down a normal life (boyfriends/girlfriends/children) is a high-wire act. And they all smoke of course; water engineers who spend their lives making clean water and dirty lungs.

There is a new plague to replace Ebola in the camp, this time from Nairobi flies. When you slap them as they bite, they release a chemical that causes a "paederus dermatitis" with nasty inflammation and blistering. I quick search of the medical literature and I find out that the Sierra Leonean versions are particularly severe. The key is to flick rather than slap when bitten, and we spend our time at the camp performing a strange chorea-form dance to each other.

On the plus side, schools have opened after a year of closure. Every school has its own isolation unit in the playground - built with simple traditional materials. I am mobbed by children when I inspect its water and sanitation facilities.

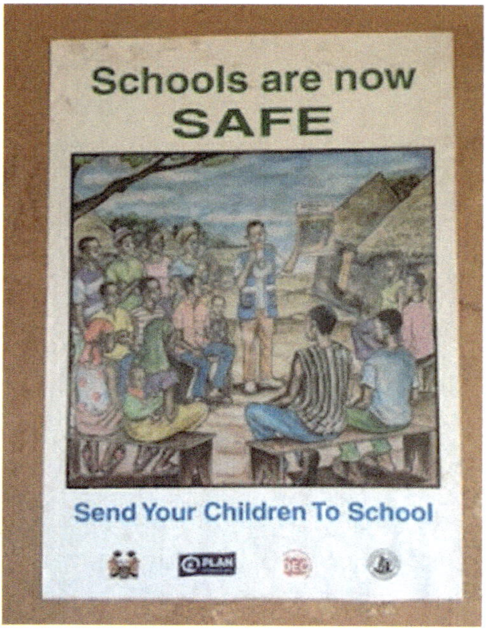

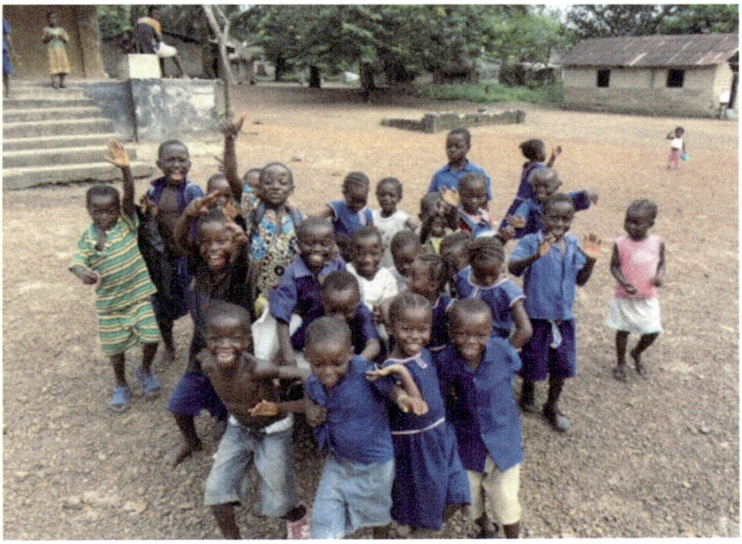

Friday, 20 November 2015
While you were gone….

Ebola has inevitably been the focus of everyone's attention in the year since I was here. But while the national and international community were away fighting the epidemic, the humdrum diseases of everyday Africa have been chomping away on their human hosts.

My colleague James Elston had undertaken a wonderful health needs assessment in Moyamba in February and I was keen to see how this had changed with the end of the epidemic. I set off on my Grand Tour of Moyamba district - like the Grand Tour of Europe, but hotter, dustier, bumpier and with fewer classical antiquities.

First stop was Moyamba Hospital where I was reunited with the impressive Dr Jonjopi who is almost single-handedly trying to keep the hospital running in the face of government apathy. They are running out of so much basic supplies (needles, gloves, scalpels, oxygen, drugs, lab kits) that I fear they may soon have to become the country's first homeopathic hospital.

The gulf in resources between our ETC and the hospital is disturbing. At the ETC we sit at our laptops in well-stocked, air-conditioned offices. Our pharmacy bulges with the latest drugs and equipment. Our supply tents are veritable Aladdins caves and outside a fleet of shiny 4x4s sit waiting to whisk us to our next destination. Yet we have no patients. Meanwhile at the hospital a battered ambulance lies rusting in the humid heat. The pharmacy cupboards are bare. The laboratory has run out of basic equipment, even needles to take blood. The ETC is the Harrods to the government hospital's car boot, and it must be galling to watch us pack up all our riches and fly it thousands of miles back to the UK when it could save many lives just down the road.

The one thing that Dr Jonjopi wants most is power. Not in an evil villain way - just electrical power. The circa 1960's generator had given up the ghost earlier in the year and now the hospital had no electricity. Meanwhile down the road at the ETC we have enough spanking new generators to light up a small European city. Even our base camp (population: 13) had two large generators.

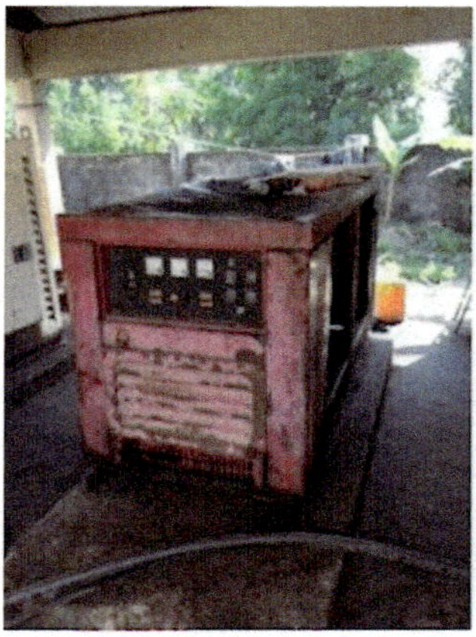
Moyamba hospital

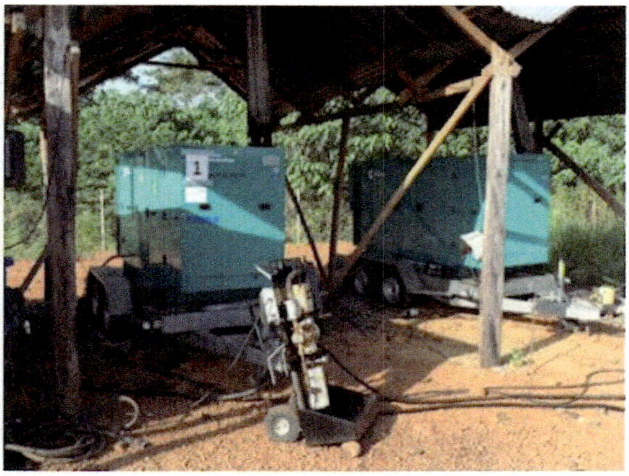
Base camp

When I was here last year I was able to requisition some of our vast mountain of DFID supplies and surreptitiously sneak them down the road to the hospital. Technically this might constitute theft from the UK tax payer, so I better keep it quiet from the GMC. However this time I am a spectator and layers of bureaucracy have grown up at the ETC like the Moyamban jungle around us, so I cannot redistribute from the rich ETC to the poor government hospital. However I promise to lobby DFID to leave one (just one itsy, bitsy generator) behind. No one will notice back home.

Dr Jonjopi has undue confidence in my ability to pull this off based on previous experience and the folklore legend that I have become in these parts, with my own nickname in the local language (Thieving Bastard Wright - it sounds much better in Mende).

Next, to a Maternal and Child Health Post - one of the basic units of the district health system, serving about 4000 people. The nurse running it was alas away on a training course (infection control!) but there were a team of three 'Ebola screeners' on guard duty to check temperatures, oversee hand washing and permit onward travel into the clinic. They wear goggles when taking my temperature which seemed a bit OTT, but assured me this is government protocol. Not quite the 'have a nice day y'all' front of house welcome I was expecting.

Then a long bumpy journey later, onto a Community Health Post, the next step up in size. It was closed. More training we were told. Note to self: do not fall acutely unwell on a training day. Onwards through the day to a Community Health Centre (the big mummy of health clinics covering 15,000 people) where we found nurses and health officers trying to hold back the tide of ill-health.

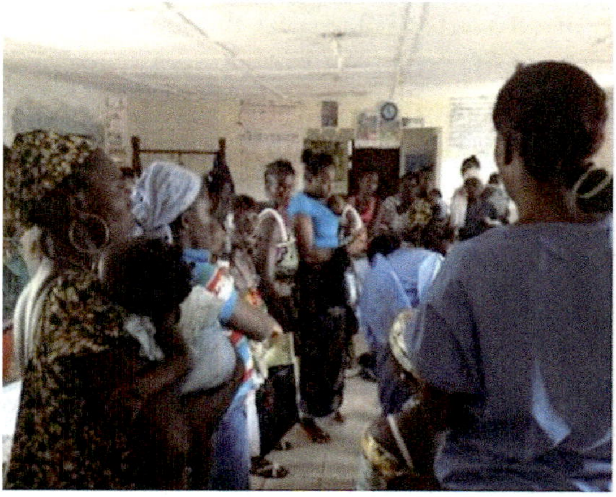
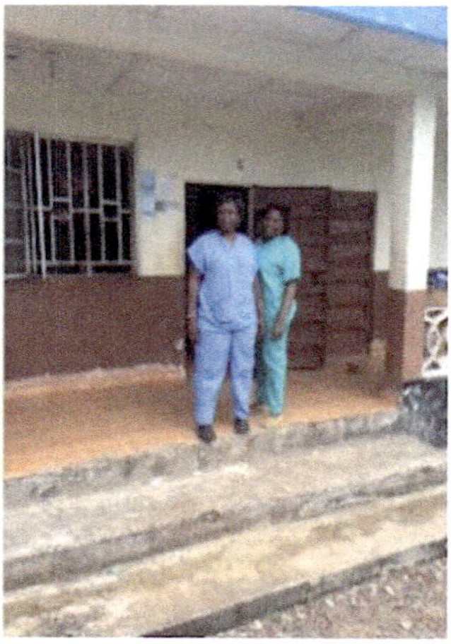

My tour continues, bagging a few more MCHPs and CHPs before my shock-absorbing back capitulates under the attack from the unmade roads and I return to the basecamp with the following conclusions:

1) People are returning to the clinics. Any fear of that these are plague centres has lifted with the end of the epidemic. However the traditional healers remain an important first point of contact.
2) The physical capital of the clinics is not bad. A bit shabby and could do with a big, slobbering lick of paint.
3) They all lack running water. Some of them have sinks and water tanks, but none of them function. This is pretty fundamental when trying to implement a ‘now wash your hands’ campaign and there is nowhere to wash them.
4) The larger clinics have a solar panel to run the single fridge that maintains the cold chain, for vaccines but like the hospital they tend to lack power.
5) Essential drugs are better stocked than I anticipated, but some basic gaps, particularly paediatric medicines, from delayed supply.
6) Rapid testing malaria, TB and HIV kits are all available. There is a shedload of malaria positive results (that’s a technical epidemiological term), but few HIV positive cases or TB positive AAFB smears. Given the level of HIV/TB in many African countries this is an encouraging sign.
7) The health workers are impressive, but a bit demotivated. Too much top down management and not enough bottom up improvement.

I suspect that the historical routine public health data that we have been using to evaluate trends in diseases is not reliable and resolve to spend tomorrow with the district surveillance team.

Saturday, 21 November 2015
They will survive

Following the Pauline Cafferkey's 'long Ebola' symptoms that were closely followed in the news, I am keen to find out what is happening with the ETCs Ebola survivors. Ebola appears to linger in our bodies after infection. Just as herpes virus lies dormant in our spinal cord after childhood chickenpox, and returns years later as a cold sore. There are 'immune privileged' sites in our body such as our eyes, spinal cord and in males, testes, that remain remote from our immune system.

The American doctor Ian Crozier recovered from Ebola to find one of his eyes changing colour from blue to green - active Ebola virus replicating in the aqueous humour of this eyeball. What a scary thought when he looked in the mirror - something out of a horror film. Pauline Cafferkey had a post-Ebola meningitis and fortunately has recovered. A paper in the New England Medical Journal found that Ebola could remain in semen for up to 9 months following infection and there has been one case at least of Ebola being sexually transmitted.

So what about our Ebola survivors? I met up with two of them. Philip (photo) and his family had all been infected with the virus. His father and two brothers had died, he and his two sisters had survived after successful care in the ETC. He had recovered fully and was now training as a community health worker so he can care for future patients, which was a wonderful completion of the circle. Mohammed had also lost members of his family and was suffering from on-going health problems and struggling to find work.

Clara is a psychologist from Madrid and runs the psychosocial team looking after around 100 local survivors. She tells me that they face two hurdles after they walk out of the happy shower at the ETC. First is the fear that they still have the virus. Some of the wives of the men have refused to have sex with them for fear of contagion of Ebola STD.

The other hurdle is acceptance back into their communities. When I was here last year the survivors I spoke to faced real stigmatisation and rejection. Their friends and neighbours were scared of catching Ebola from them. This has changed dramatically over recent months. The end of Ebola has helped of course, but education and awareness and contact has overcome the prejudice. A powerful example of overcoming discrimination in society.

A weak link in the chain for many of them is the loss of other family members. The nature of Ebola meant that it tends to effect clusters in close contact. Many of the survivors were struggling with the loss of their family support network, and perhaps survivor guilt.

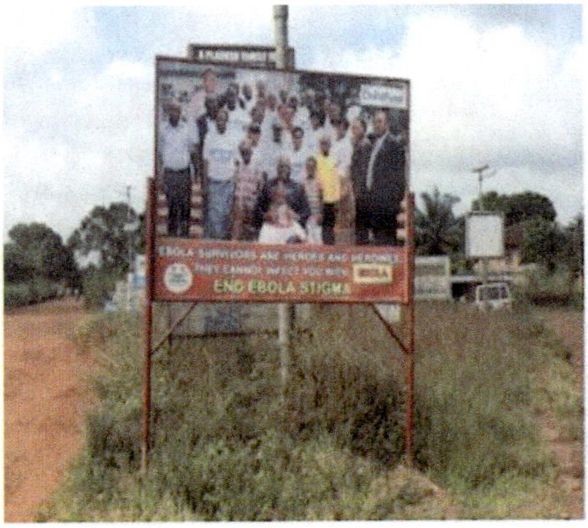
END EBOLA STIGMA

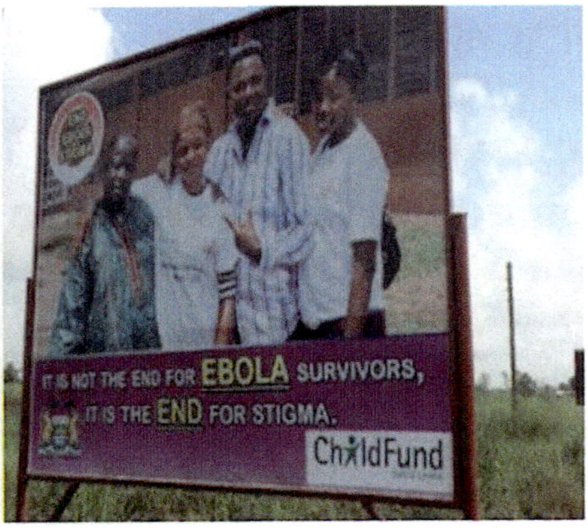
IT IS NOT THE END FOR EBOLA SURVIVORS,
IT IS THE END FOR STIGMA.
ChildFund

They are still collecting the data on sequelae, but the preliminary data suggests that about 50% of patients have on-going physical symptoms - uveitis is common, joint pains (bilateral, affecting upper and lower limbs) and headache. Some have experienced hair loss. There do not appear to have been any serious complications such as meningitis, but some of the patients do live in very remote areas, so keeping track of them can be a challenge.

Last month the team managed to get 90 of the survivors together for a celebration last month. It was a special occasion - much dancing and singing. All members of a very special club: they saw Ebola and lived.

I return to the Ebola cemetery on the outskirts of town. The last time I was here was to arrange a burial for one of our first patients. There were a dozen grave diggers in full PPE sweating away in the heat to dig the deep Ebola graves. This time the place is deserted, but the number of grave markers has grown to hundreds. It is a beautiful and tranquil resting place and I suspect within a year will be overtaken by the jungle and return completely to nature. However it will always be a memorial to those who were not lucky enough to survive.

Monday, 23 November 2015
Something for the weekend

The weekend has been reclaimed from Ebola-work with a rest day on Sunday. However three new cases in Liberia after nearly two months of Ebola-freedom jolts us from the celebratory complacency. Like the fight against IS, the fight with Ebola is asymmetric warfare, striking when we least expect it.

There is a national Thanksgiving Day for the end of Ebola and Moyamba does its bit by holding a multi faith celebration. Around half the population is Muslim and half Christian - living together in a model of peace and mutual respect. Community leaders gather at the Ebola Response Centre to give thanks. The 9am start stretches and yawns to mid-morning when proceedings finally kick off.

Europeans have lost the art of public speaking. We are too self-conscious in our aim to get across the key messages. Too nervous to do without powerpoint or autocue. Africans in contrast can hold an audience for hours with their narrative skills, and we sit in awe of the Moyamban loquaciousness but also vain hope that they might revert to bullet points.

The Christian community leader starts off with a praise-the-lord thanks for the end of Ebola, but his oratory soon deteriorates into comparisons with Sodom and Gomorrah and God's punishment for homosexuality. Ebola has been the Lord's punishment for all our terrible, debauched sinning he cries out, scanning the room until his gaze finally settles firmly on me. I freeze. How the feck does he know?
The weekend is also the time for the Premier league and a chance to live show off local passion for English football. Man United is the most popular team, followed by Arsenal, Liverpool and Chelsea. Saturday afternoon find everyone sitting around TV screens watching all the live matches. No Sky subscriptions needed in Moyamba. Every time a goal is scored, wild celebrations break out with shouting and laps of honour round the room - more exuberant celebrations than the on-screen goal-scorers.

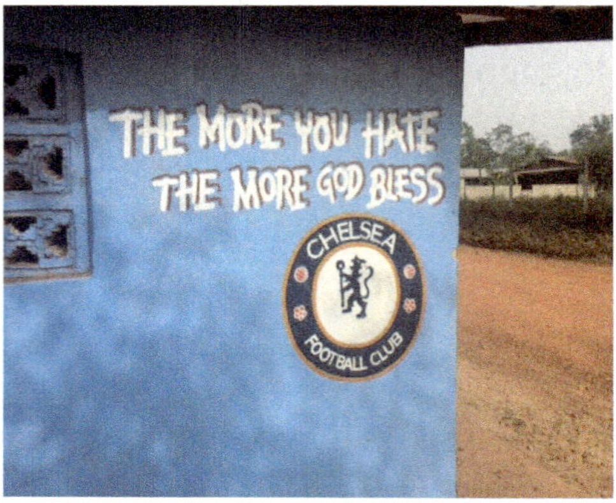
THE MORE YOU HATE
THE MORE GOD BLESS
CHELSEA
FOOTBALL CLUB

The base camp has been finally abandoned. We have all been moved to a guest house in town, exchanging our shared air-conditioned tents with cramped, shared, non-air-conditioned rooms that become sweltering saunas in the night. The lack of sleep sparks an atmosphere of irritability made worse by the disruption to our twice daily addiction to the peanut-chicken-rice staple diet.

The ETC is also coming down around us. There are also an increasing number of thefts going on despite the G4S security guards (or perhaps because of). Yesterday it was 14 mattresses. Mattresses? Not the sort of thing that you stick down your trousers as you walk past the guards. Let them have it all is my view - better to leave all this Ebola bounty to local people than whisk it back to the UK where second-hand Ebola mattresses are unlikely to meet their asking price on Ebola Ebay.

The district health team want to take over the solid buildings at the Centre, but I am not convinced this is such a great move. Despite the skill of the Royal Engineers, this is not a place that will survive the ages, even months. Next to the Chinese factory making iPads for demanding Californians, is a factory making stuff for Africa, and it is crap. Yesterday one of the French aid workers flushed the toilet and the whole cistern, bowel and pipes shattered and collapsed, leaving her left holding just the metal handle with nothing attached to it.

It is a message from God. The one that the Christian community leader follows. I pack my bags and head to Freetown. My work here is done.

I will miss Moyamba. Everywhere I go people shout "Doctor John' in a sing-song greeting, laughing and waving. They may be laughing at me, but I don't care. I love the joy of it, and might introduce it as a compulsory greeting for my team in Bradford. As I leave the ETC for the final time the guard at the entrance hugs me and points out that I was the first doctor in and the last doctor out. Like a party guest that you just can't get rid of.

Wednesday, 25 November 2015
It's all about the money

Ebola is evil and of course money is the root of it, and its enduring impact. The lack of investment in the public health infrastructure following its decimation during the civil war, both in Sierra Leone and Liberia, undoubtedly contributed to the spread of the epidemic through poor urban communities with little access to clean water. The World Bank estimates the international community spent $2 billion on the emergency Ebola response. A fraction of this invested after the civil war would have gone a long way to preventing the outbreak and saving a huge amount of money. Prevention is better, and cheaper than the cure, but it's the headline-grabbing treatment that tends to persuade the public and politicians.

Sierra Leone is 183rd in the UN Development Index, and Liberia a lofty 175th, out of 187 countries. The main industries of tourism and mining scarpered at the first sign of Ebola. The tourists are reportedly starting to trickle back, but I didn't see many sombreros and Hawaiian shirts at the airport - all the white people had 'aid worker' written (often literally) all over them. The mines are also starting to open, but the price of iron has plummeted apparently and many remain closed.

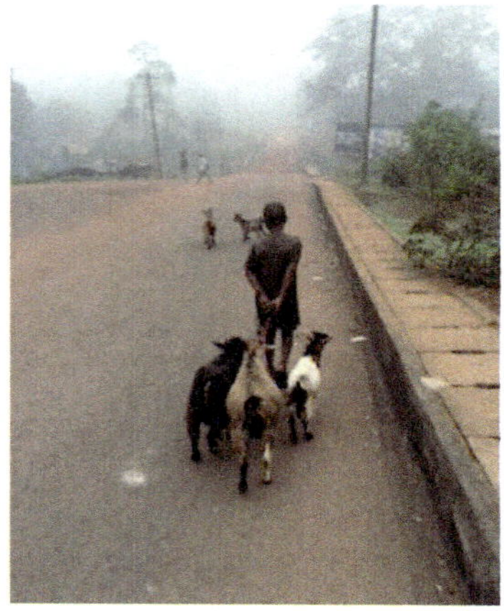

It is a fertile country with great mineral wealth and Bounty-advert beaches, so the potential is there, and if there was a hedge fund trade on the UN Development Index it would be good bet to place money on economic improvement.

Moyamba itself looks as though little has changed since the Victorians were here. Outside of the town it looks as though little has changed since biblical times. There are few jobs and subsistence farming is the mainstay of survival. The daily chores of carrying water from the well, washing and fetching firewood are done swith sense of community and bonding.

On the plus side levels of inequality are low - everyone is poor. And no one around here is overweight - a simple diet and the physical activity of daily routines keeps everyone fit. And people seem pretty happy. I am struck by the contrast most when I travel back from a rural African town to the UK. One day I can be at the centre of TB/HIV/Ebola epidemics, but I will stand in the main street and marvel at the laughter and love that fills the dusty air. A few hours later I will be travelling through London with the grim-faced commuters. Actually, it's not all about the money.

There has been an Ebola dividend in Moyamba. Large amounts of money have flowed into the town to build the ETC and then create precious jobs - hundreds of them. People have been happy to take on high risk jobs that come with a danger supplement. But now they are all being made redundant and the future is dim. Perversely most of the ETC would rather the epidemic continues so that they are able to maintain an income.

At a national level, as is depressingly common in Africa, there has inevitably been corruption and profiteering from the huge amounts of aid money that have flowed into the country. I meet a Wold Bank official who candidly admits that of the $2 billion in aid, probably about half remains unaccounted for. A small number of senior politicians and officials will have squirreled away unimaginable sums of money in off-shore bank accounts.

At a smaller scale I loved the story from one of my French colleagues about recycled vehicles. The British government has imported over a hundred pickup trucks to support the emergency response. My French colleague was part of a NGO distributing and maintaining them. To his great surprise the brand new vehicles started breaking down within a week. When they investigated more closely they found that they had been completed stripped down and rebuilt with old parts, the original parts spirited away to refresh the local transport fleets. Such ingenuity and *cajones*.

Thursday 25 November 2015

I am back in Freetown, luxuriating in a room at the Seaside View - my own room, running water and electricity. Food that is not peanut-chicken-rice. I sleep more hours in my first night than the entire previous week.

The hotel lives up to its name by providing a view of the sea. It is one of a row of similar tours hotels lining the rocky Atlantic shore. All of them completely deserted. I look out over an abandoned hotel extension: a throw-back to more optimistic times. Chinese factory ships trawl up and down the sea lanes offshore - making fish while the sun shines. Making a lot of fish while the sun shines, and with no local coast guard to enforce territorial waters.

I join the mad dogs in the heat and explore my neighbours. A giant international conference centre stands forlorn and empty. Idris the security guard of a nearby hotel invites me in to admire the marble and mezzanine. I feel I am a sole survivor in a post-apocalyptic world.

I pass three men toiling in the heat with make-do hammers. On one end of their production line they have large boulders and on the other small stones. their unenviable task is to break rocks in the hot sun, producing progressively smaller pebbles. It seems like a Sisyphean task, one more appropriate for a machine, and I wonder about its purpose - building materials I guess.

Friday 25 November 2015

It's time to go home. Flights have returned to some normality though the plane is half empty and I get a rare upgrade to business class which makes the disparity of wealth from where I have come in Moyamba painfully acute. But turning down free champagne and reclining seats seems a bit of a pointless hair-shirted stance to take so I indulge myself.

At Heathrow there are no chaotic scenes from a year ago. No public health screening teams or media scrum. I make my way to Kings Cross and the train north to home, reflective as always when returning from a trip to Africa. A bit of me has changed forever, a bit of me more angry at the global inequality that I have experienced, a bit of me more grateful for my accident of (global North) birth, and a bit of me more determined to try harder to make a difference. I know from experience that my new zeal will wash away rapidly in the whitewater of our consumer society, but for now I cherish it and the promise it holds.

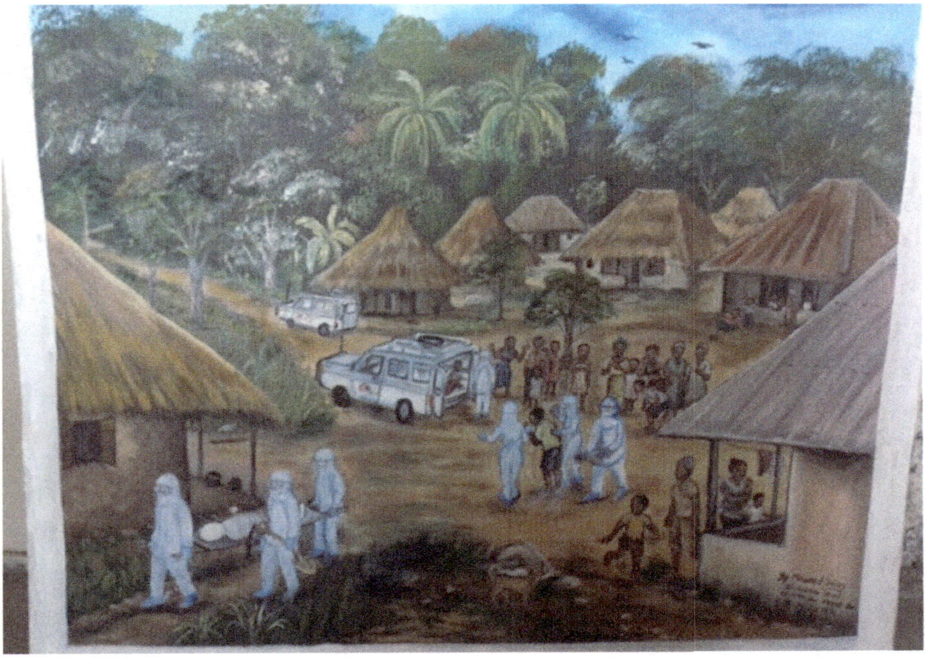

Epilogue

West Africa was safe, but over the following years small fires of Ebola ignited across the Democratic Republic of Congo. The West African epidemic had focused the minds of scientists (and funders). There is little profit to be made in the treatment of tropical illnesses as they present in countries that cannot afford new and expensive medicines. However and after many years of neglect a number of hopeful treatments have been developed in preparation for the next outbreak. Crucially, simple and rapid diagnostic PCR tests have been developed that will speed up detection and isolation.

In 2021 the virus returned to Guinea in a small cluster and then Ivory Coast for the first time in almost 30 years. By that time the rest of the world was pre-occupied by another virus.

When I first read about Covid19 in the medical journals my 25 years of experience started jumping up and down in alarm. This was clearly something different. A highly infectious disease that was spreading rapidly, not confined to poor countries but on the march. It was coming at exponential speed: first gradually and then very suddenly.

African countries affected by infectious disease outbreaks have learnt harsh lessons and prepared in earnest for the next inevitable epidemic. In Europe we have become blasé about communicable disease – it is something that happens in foreign lands to poor people. I never imagined that I would ever be applying my Ebola experience to Bradford. In March 2020 as we watched with fear and uncertainty as the tsunami hurtled towards us, I assumed there would be plans and preparedness for this sort of event. Such optimism was quickly dispelled as my hospital filled with sick and dying patients and we scrabbled about to find PPE and testing capacity.

We tend to have a paternalistic attitude to medicine inn Africa. The direction of knowledge flow is always from the rich North to the poor South. My own experience taught me how invaluable the lessons I learnt in African hospitals were for my NHS practice, and when it came to tackling Covid19 this had never been so true.

I found myself training staff for donning and doffing PPE (who would have thought this three letter acronym would become such a part of the national vocabulary?). Designing red zones and green zones on old NHS hospital wards that were just not built for effective isolation. I was able to understand the importance of community engagement and anticipate the waves of false news and loss of trust. Joining the District Gold Command for daily sit-reps and planning.

We will learn our lesson this time. As Eisenhower famously said, 'plans are useless but planning is indispensable'. As with Africa the large variation in death rates from COVID19 across socio-economic and ethnic groups has brought into sharp relief the inequalities in our society and the underlying distribution of risk factors for and high levels of chronic disease. The pandemic has highlighted this gap between the rich and poor in our own country, just as Ebola did between the global South and North.

As we move into post-pandemic recovery we have a unique opportunity to intervene intensively and effectively to mitigate some of the added disadvantage caused by the response to the pandemic and more generally build a better future that recognises the connectedness in our global village and the unfair distribution of the burden of disease.

Acknowledgements

To all the staff and community in Moyamba: I have such immense respect for the quiet dedication and commitment that has endured through civil war and epidemics. Such personal triumph from such challenging adversity. To Helen for her patience and support as I upped and left at such short notice. A deep debt of gratitude to Carolyn Clover who pulled my random musings into a coherent whole. To Chris Bulstrode for his wisdom and companionship and to Sue Mitchell for her magical BBC radio production.

About the author

John Wright, a doctor and epidemiologist, is head of the Bradford Institute for Health Research, and a veteran of cholera, HIV and Ebola epidemics in sub-Saharan Africa. For more information visit www.docjohnwright.com or follow him @docjohnwright

Printed in Great Britain
by Amazon

12102277R00098